BACK to SCHOOL
CORONAVIRUS
HEALTH & SAFETY ACTIVITIES

FOR KINDERGARTEN AND FIRST GRADE

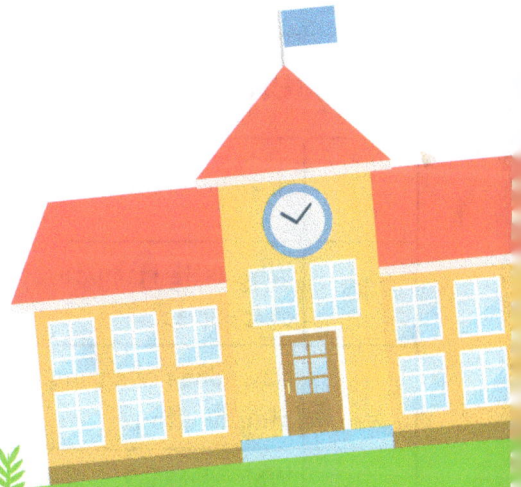

*PLEASE CONSULT YOUR LOCAL AUTHORITIES ABOUT THE LATEST RESEARCH AND SAFETY MEASURES ADVISED BY HEALTH PROFESSIONALS. CERTAIN MEASURES, SUCH AS WEARING A MASK, MAY NOT BE SUITABLE FOR CHILDREN OF CERTAIN AGES.

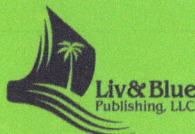

Liv&Blue
Publishing, LLC

Record of Learning

The Coronavirus

4	Why is it called coronavirus, and what does COVID-19 mean?	😀 🙂 😕 😬
6	What is a virus?	😀 🙂 😕 😬
8	How does a virus spread in my body?	😀 🙂 😕 😬
10	How does a virus spread from one person to another?	😀 🙂 😕 😬
12	What are the signs that I or someone else might be sick?	😀 🙂 😕 😬

Prevention Behavior

14	How do I know if I'm keeping enough social distance?	😀 🙂 😕 😬
16	Why is it risky to spend time in a large crowd of people?	😀 🙂 😕 😬
18	How does wearing a mask help me or others stay healthy?	😀 🙂 😕 😬
20	Why shouldn't I hug my friends or shake other people's hands?	😀 🙂 😕 😬
22	Why shouldn't we share our writing utensils and other materials?	😀 🙂 😕 😬
24	How could I get sick from touching my face?	😀 🙂 😕 😬
26	How does airing out a room reduce the risk of getting sick?	😀 🙂 😕 😬

Sanitation

28	What should I do if I have to cough or sneeze?	😀 😊 😕 😖
30	How should I wash my hands so they're clean enough?	😀 😊 😕 😖
32	Does hand sanitizer work as well as washing with soap and water?	😀 😊 😕 😖

Nutrition

| 34 | How does drinking water help my body fight viruses and sickness? | 😀 😊 😕 😖 |
| 36 | Which foods keep me healthy? | 😀 😊 😕 😖 |

Physical Health

38	Why are sports, exercise and other physical activities good for me?	😀 😊 😕 😖
40	What games can I play with my friends if I have to keep social distance?	😀 😊 😕 😖
42	How much sleep should I get every night to stay healthy?	😀 😊 😕 😖

Keep a record of your learning and reflect on your experiences! How did each activity make you feel?

😀 Great! This was a lot of fun and I learned so much!

😊 Good. This was pretty interesting and I understood it.

😕 So-so. This was a little hard but I learned something.

😖 Bad. This was hard and I still don't understand it.

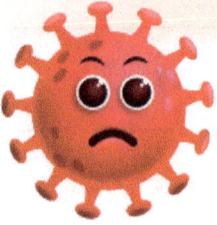

WHY IS IT CALLED CORONAVIRUS, AND WHAT DOES COVID-19 MEAN?

Connect the numbered dots and color the shape red. Then connect the lettered dots and color the shape yellow.

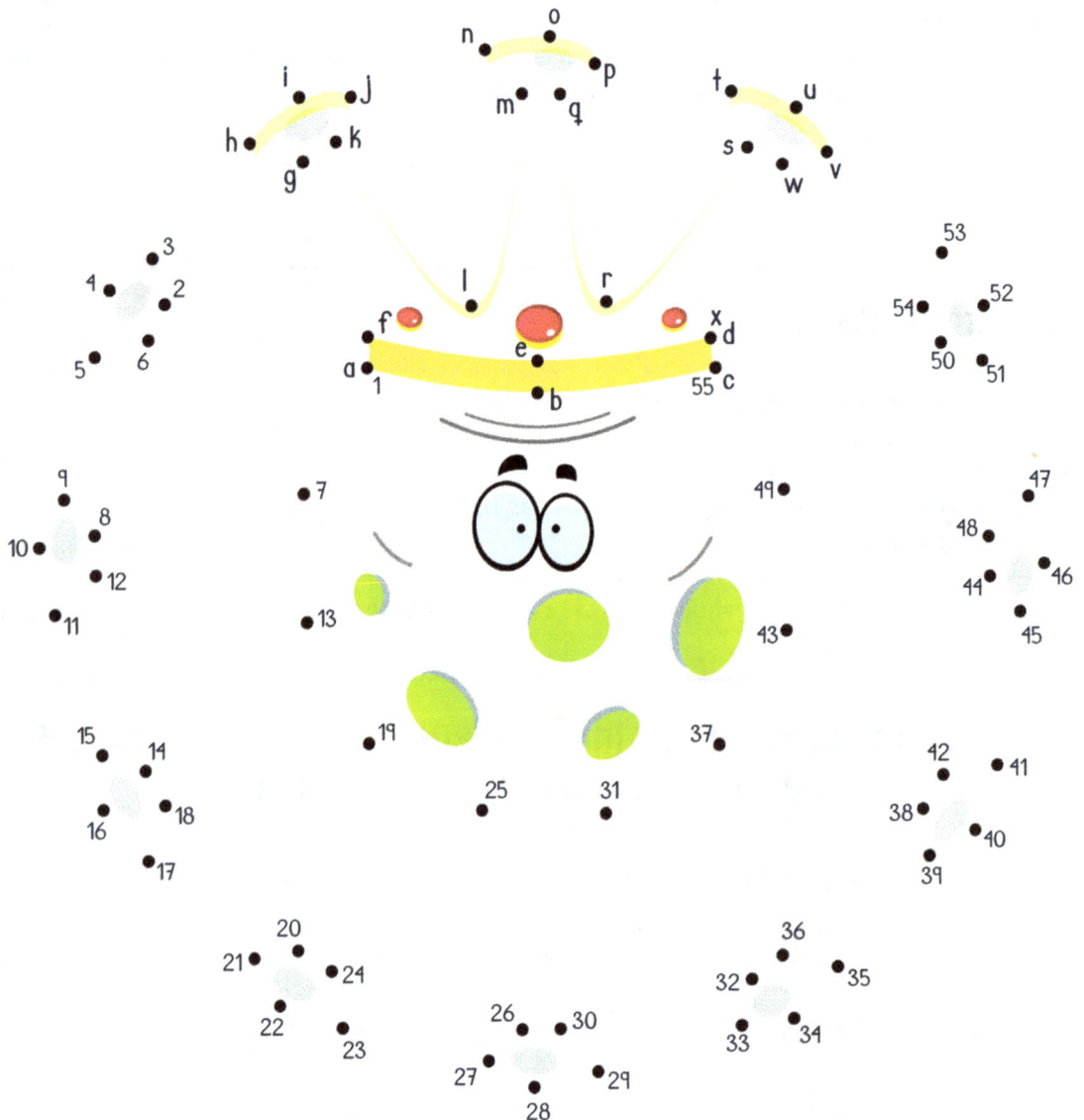

Complete the puzzle by coloring in the missing pieces and writing the letters inside.

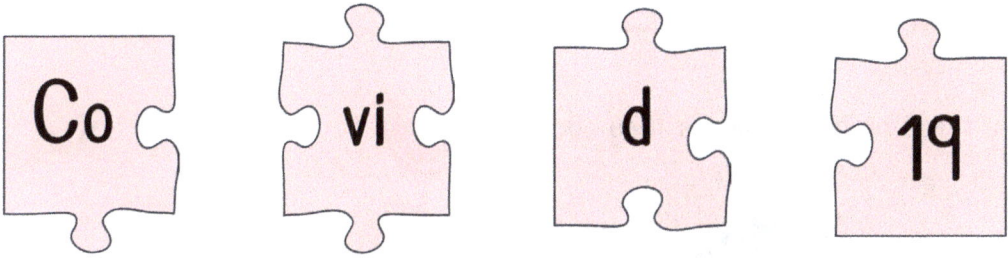

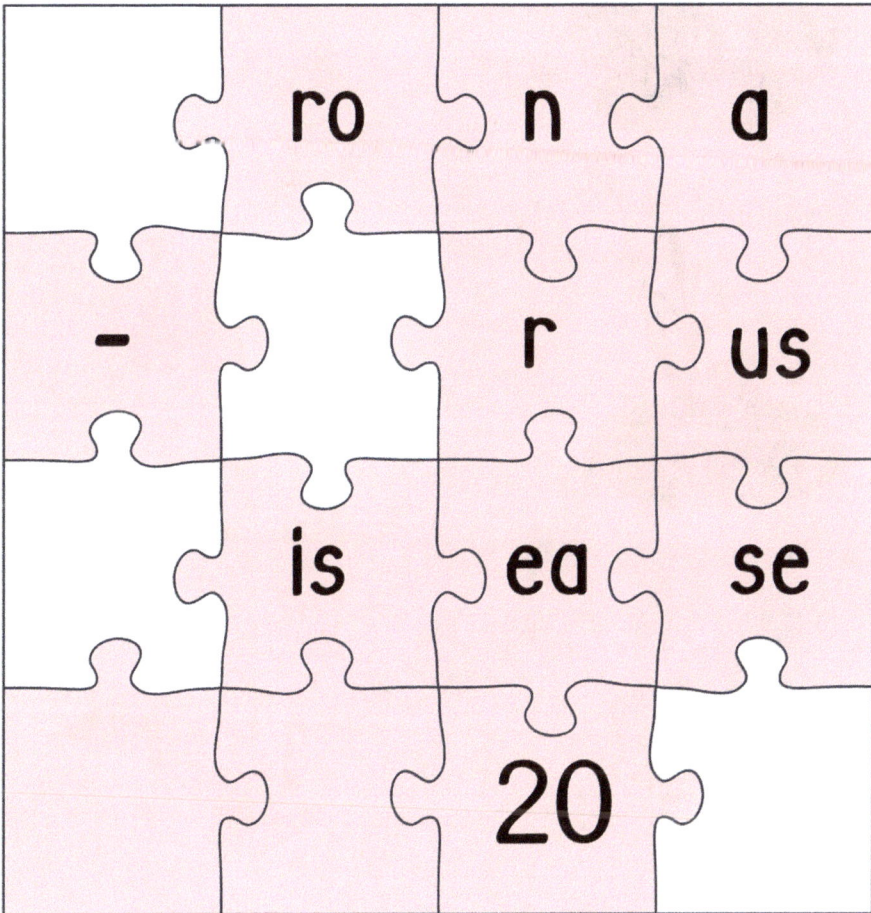

Co   vi   d   19

ro   n   a

-         r   us

is   ea   se

20

The virus looks like a **crown**, and **crown** in Latin is **corona**. COVID-19 is the name for the disease the virus causes: **Co** (corona) **vi** (virus) **D** (disease) -19 (discovered in 2019).

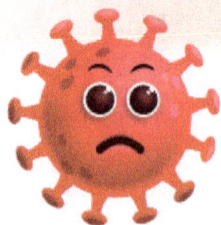

What is a virus?

Draw seeds on all the places they can grow.

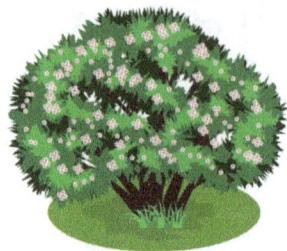

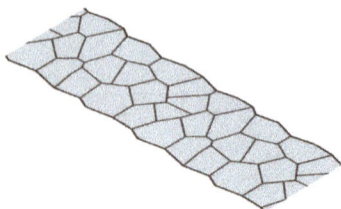

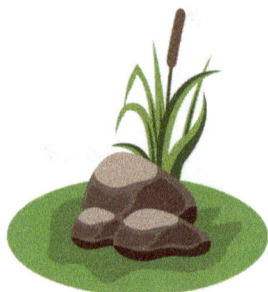

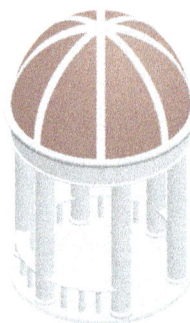

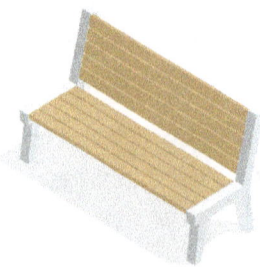

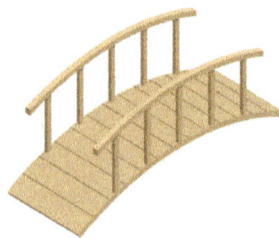

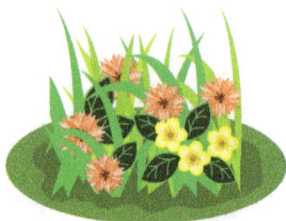

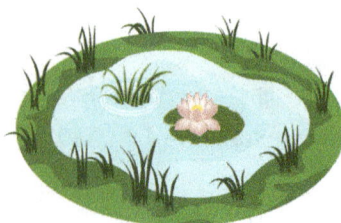

Draw viruses on all the places they can grow.

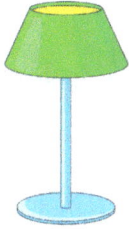

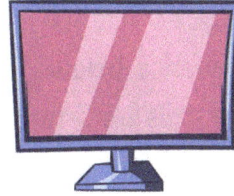

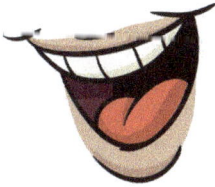

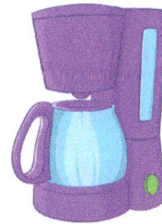

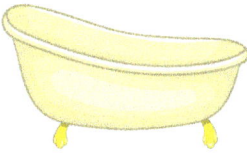

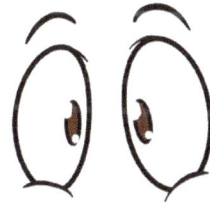

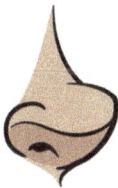

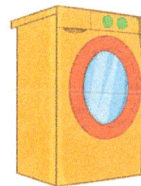

A virus is a germ somewhere in between living and nonliving, like a seed. In the right places it can grow, but it cannot grow all by itself. It needs the cells in our bodies to reproduce.

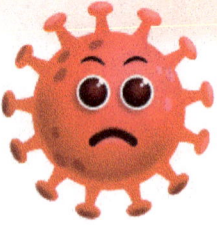

HOW DOES A VIRUS SPREAD IN MY BODY?

Look at the sequence below. Then on the next page show how viruses can multiply and infect more cells by drawing the missing pictures in the white boxes.

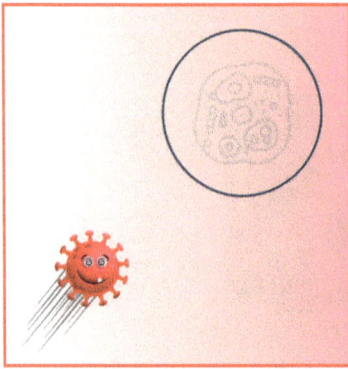

1. Virus finds cell.

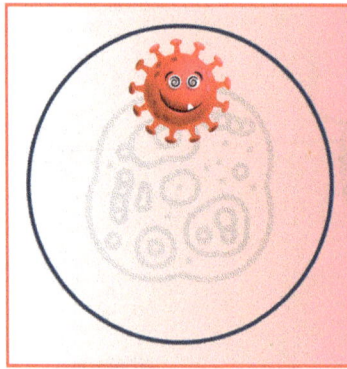

2. Virus enters cell.

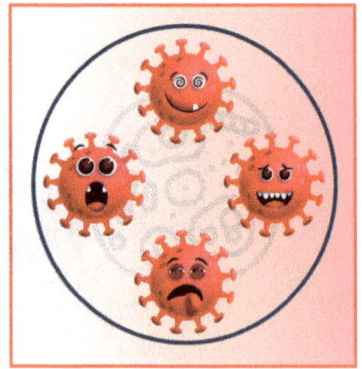

3. Virus makes copies of itself in cell.

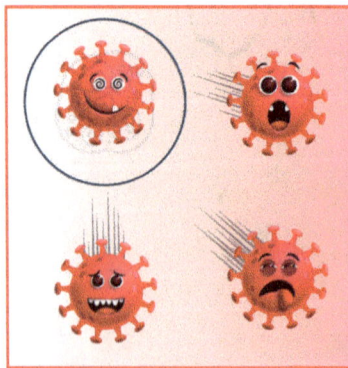

4. New viruses leave cell.

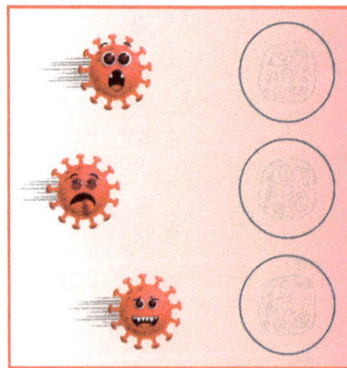

5. New viruses find other cells.

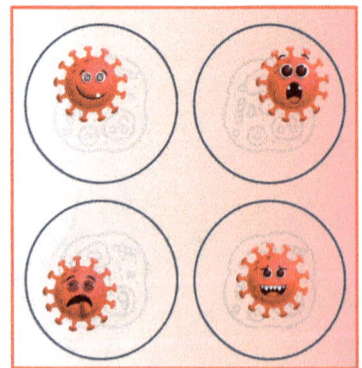

6. New viruses enter other cells....

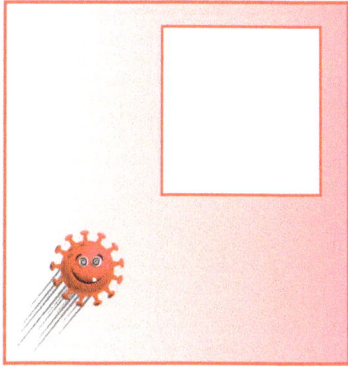

1. Virus finds cell.

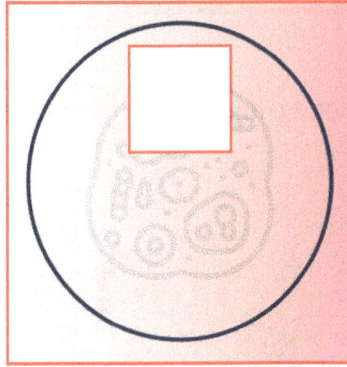

2. Virus enters cell.

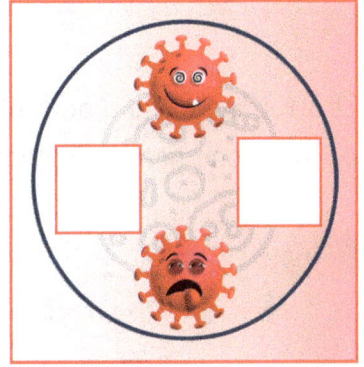

3. Virus makes copies of itself in cell.

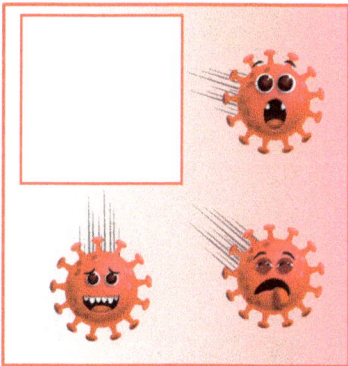

4. New viruses leave cell.

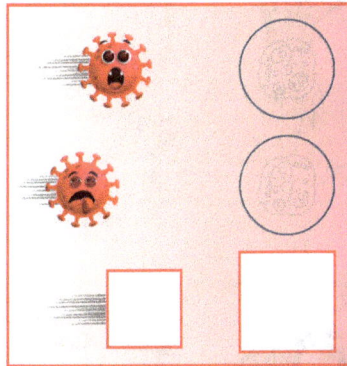

5. New viruses find other cells.

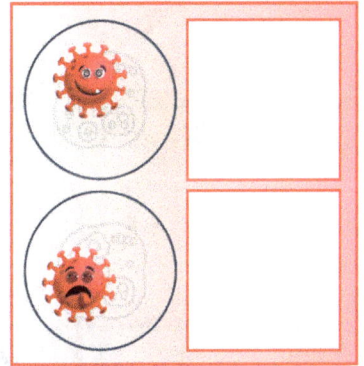

6. New viruses enter other cells....

A virus spreads by making copies of itself inside a cell and releasing these copies into your body to invade more cells and make more copies.

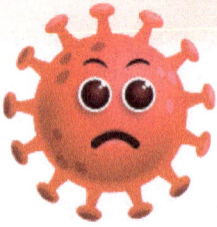

How does a virus spread from one person to another?

Draw a line along a path of hands, noses, mouths and eyes that a virus could travel on from one person to another.

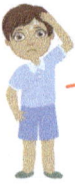

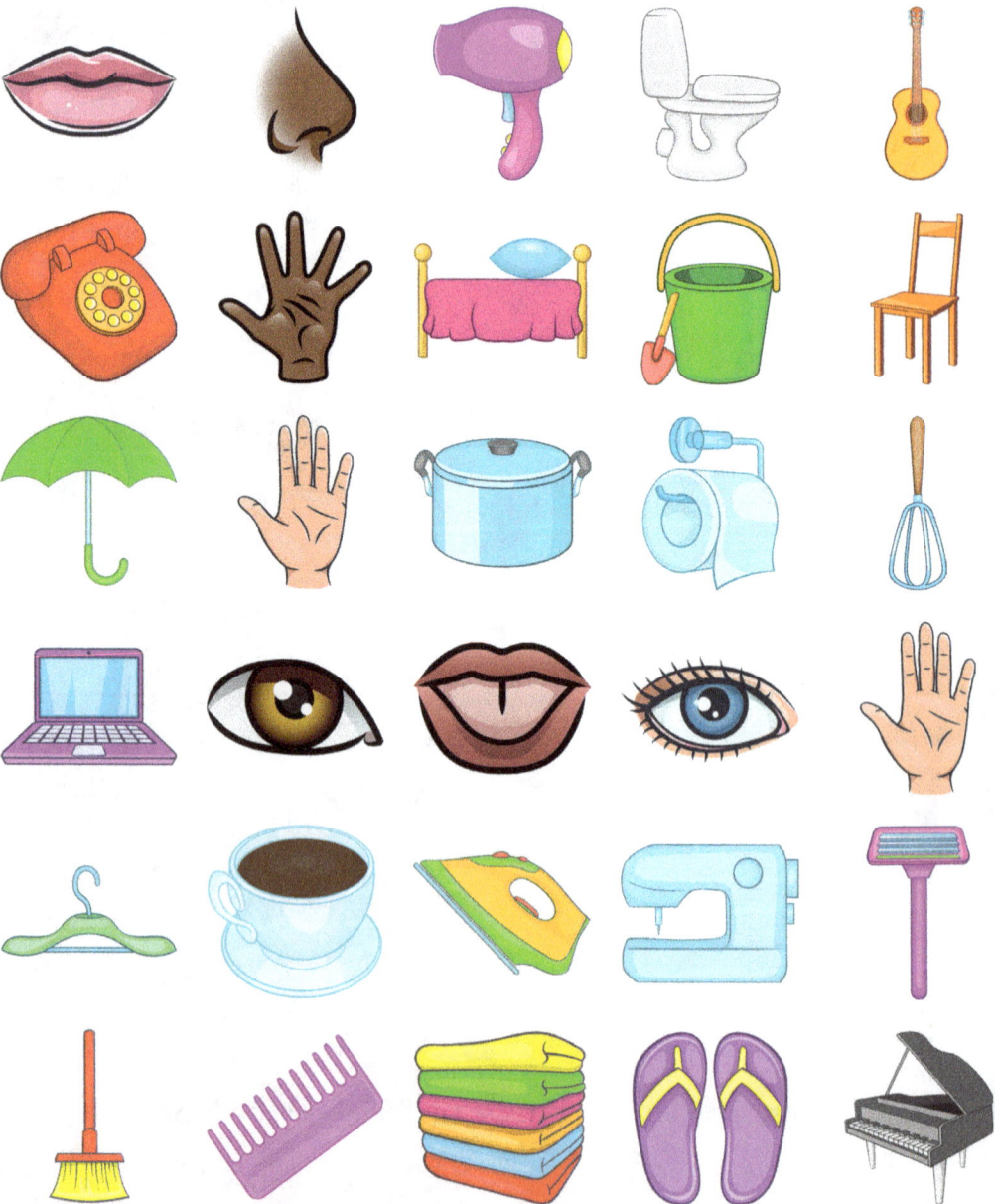

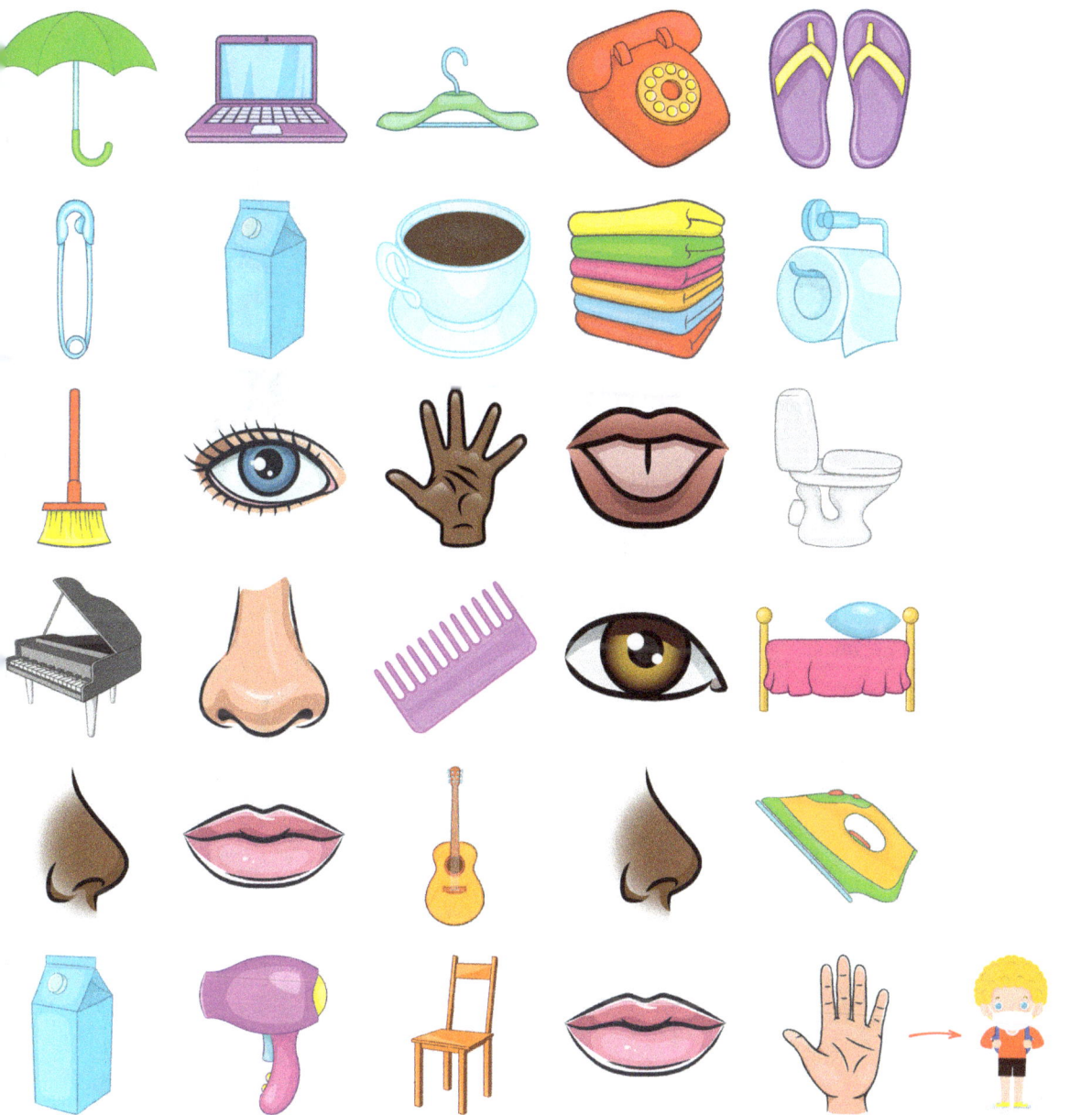

The coronavirus often infects our lungs, so it can fly out through a cough or a sneeze and travel into someone else's lungs if they touch it or breathe it in.

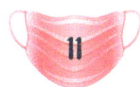

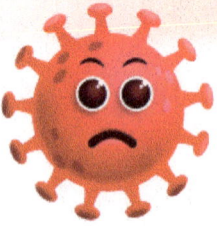

WHAT ARE THE SIGNS THAT I OR SOMEONE ELSE MIGHT BE SICK?

Circle all the kids who might be sick.

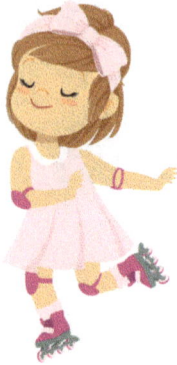

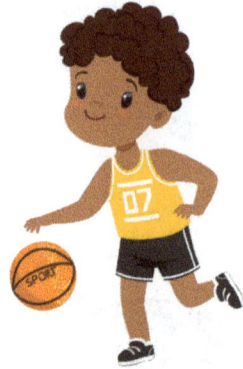

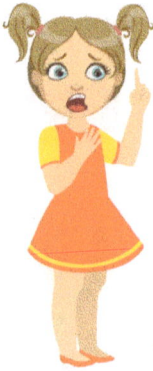

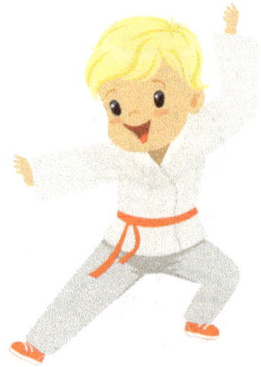

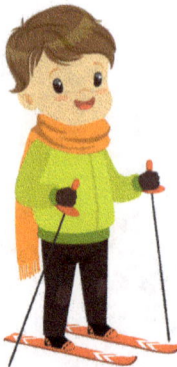

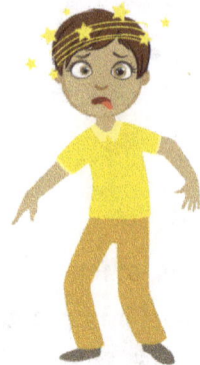

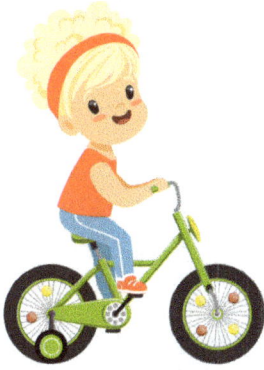

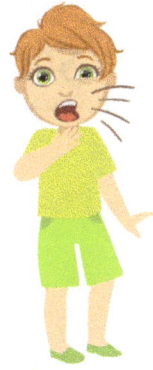

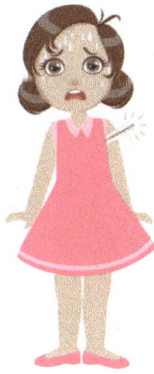

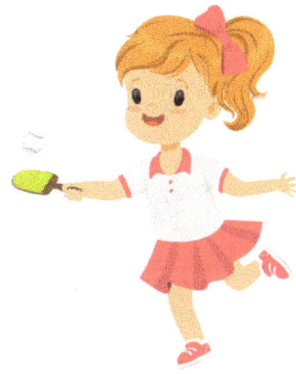

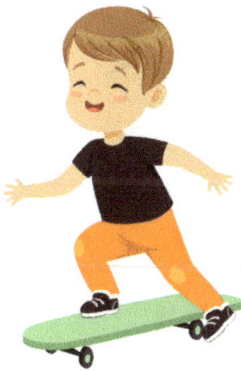

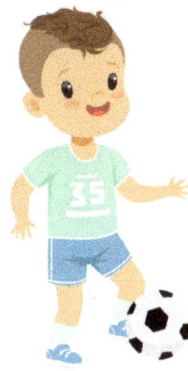

Some symptoms of the disease include coughing, fever, headache, or sore throat. If you feel sick, stay home from school.

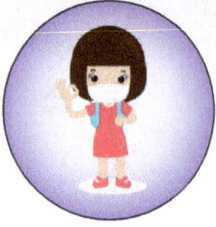

How do I know if I'm keeping enough social distance?

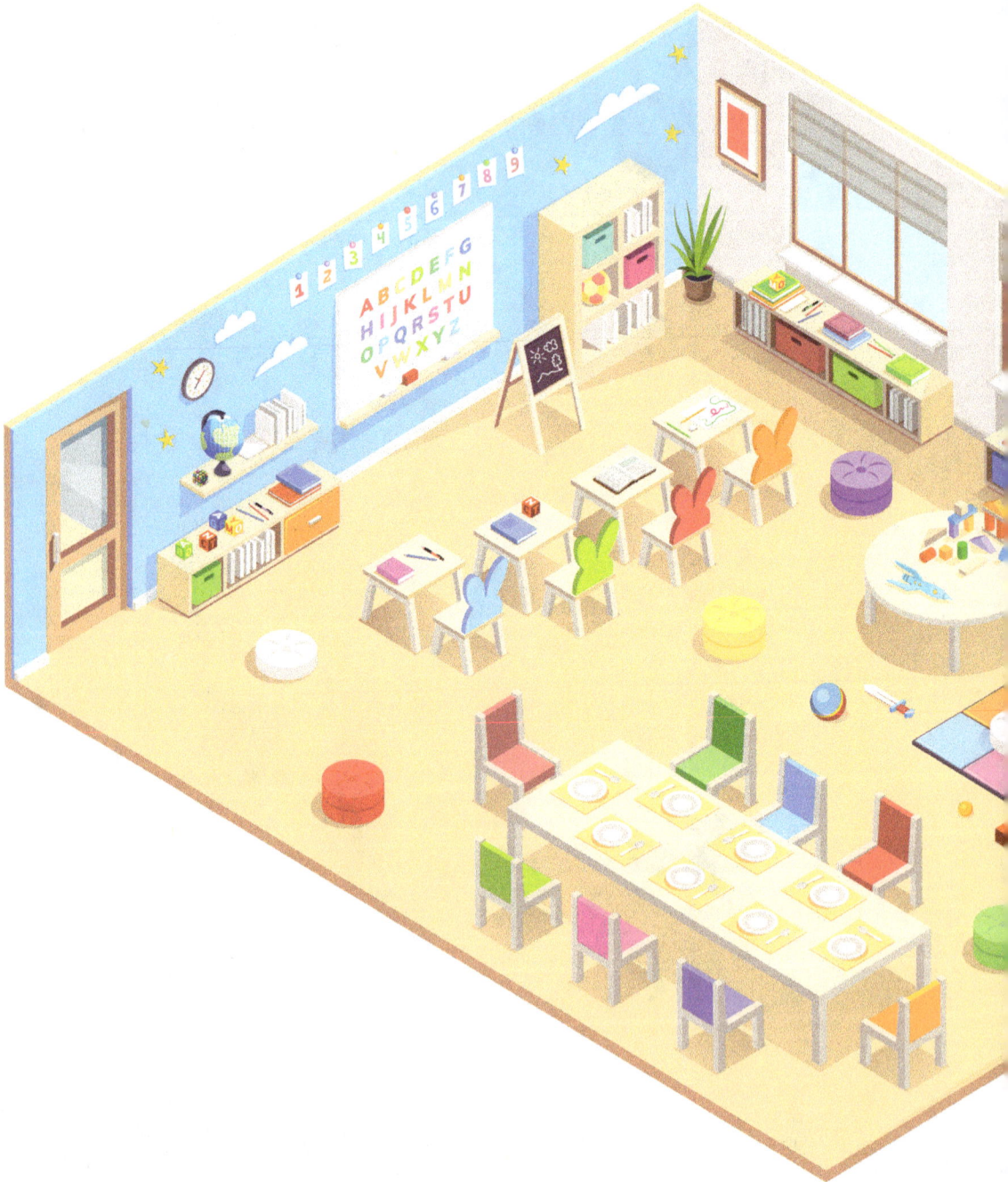

Draw some of your friends and yourself learning in this classroom while keeping enough distance between each other.

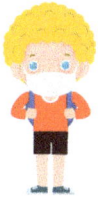

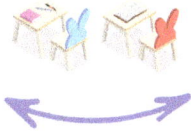

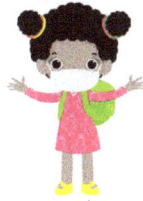

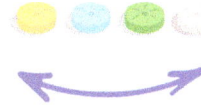

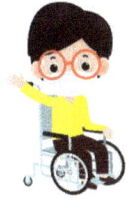

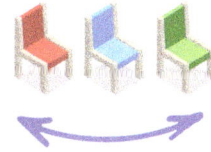

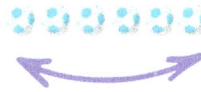

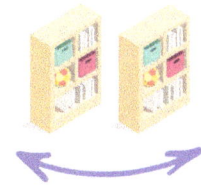

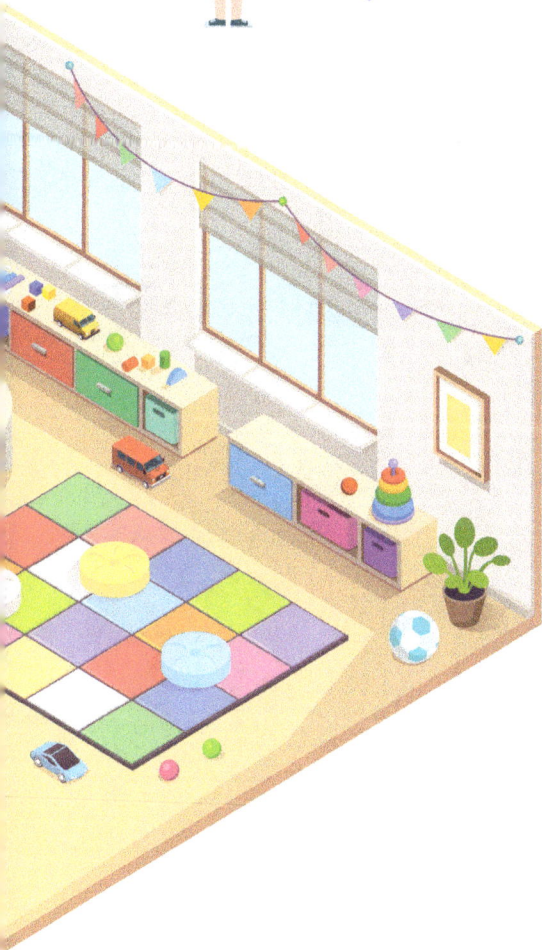

Common social distancing suggestions include 6 feet or 1.5 meters. Imagining an object this length between you and your friends will help keep you safely apart.

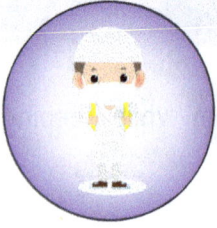

WHY IS IT RISKY TO SPEND TIME IN A LARGE CROWD OF PEOPLE?

Shade in as many children's shapes as you can without overlapping colors.

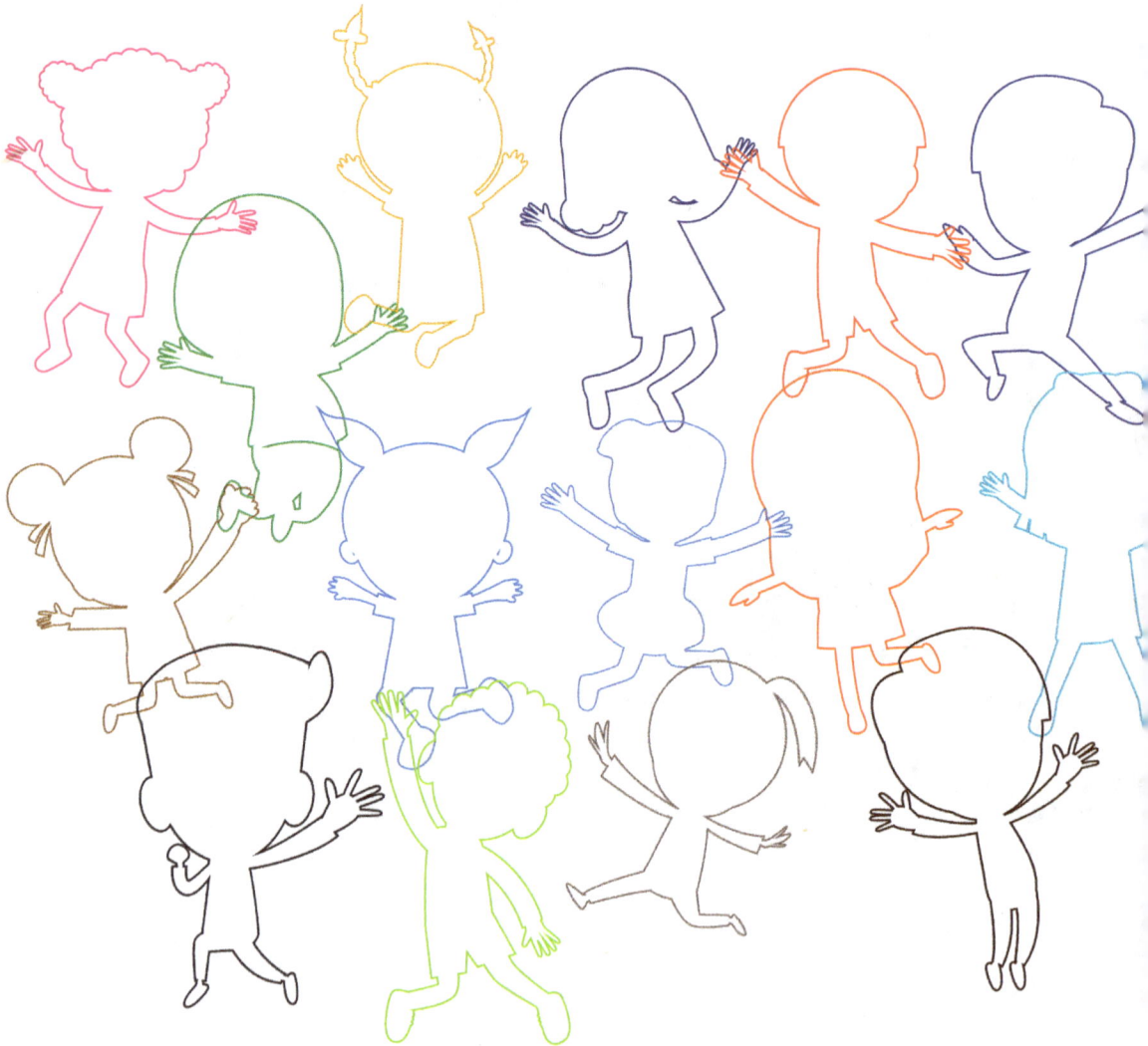

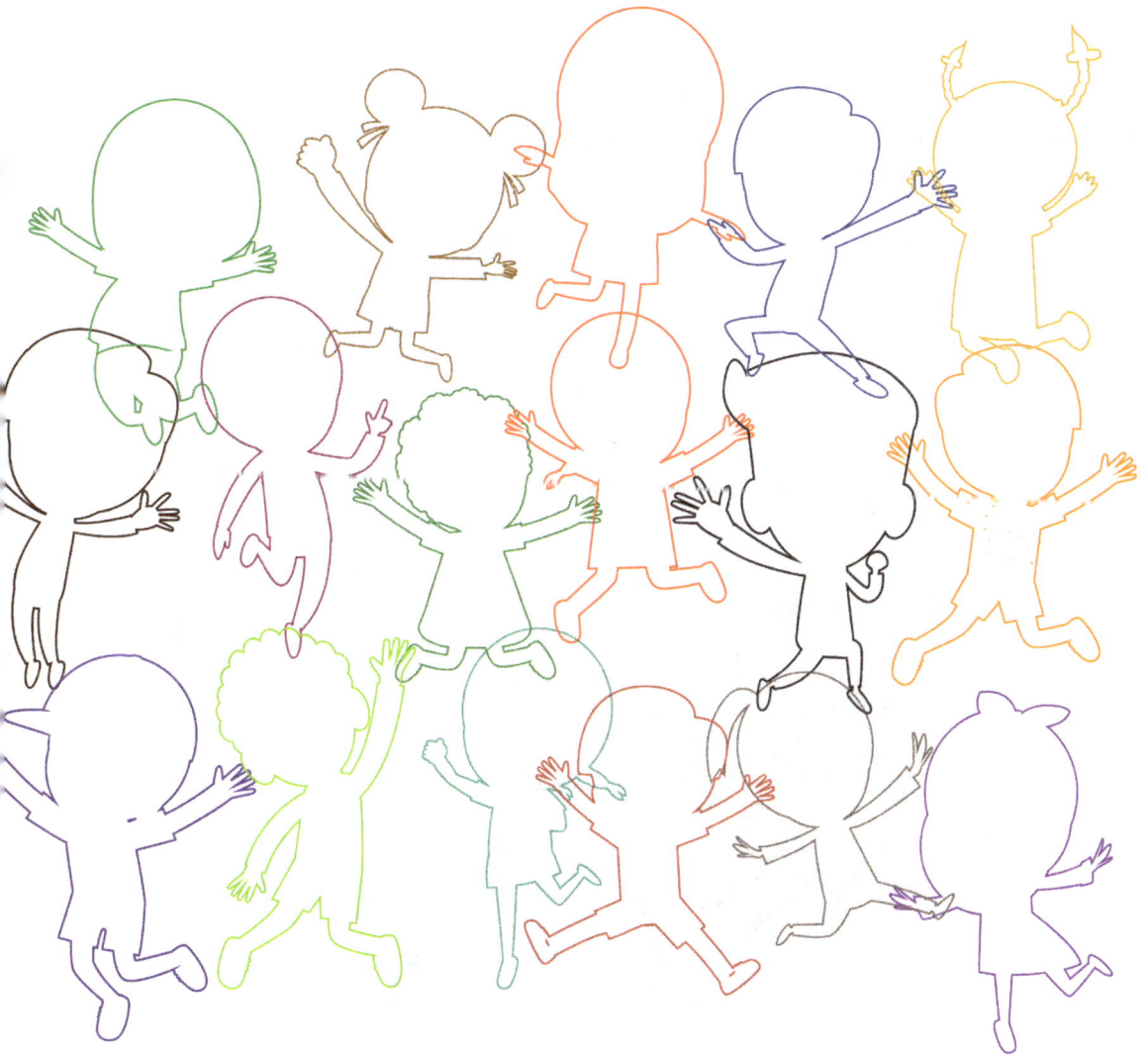

Coronavirus spreads to people, from people. The more people in a group, the greater the chance someone might be sick. Avoiding crowds = avoiding sickness.

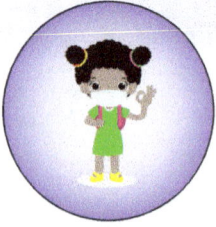

HOW DOES WEARING A MASK HELP ME OR OTHERS STAY HEALTHY?

Help the virus find its way out of the mouth, only to get caught by the mask.

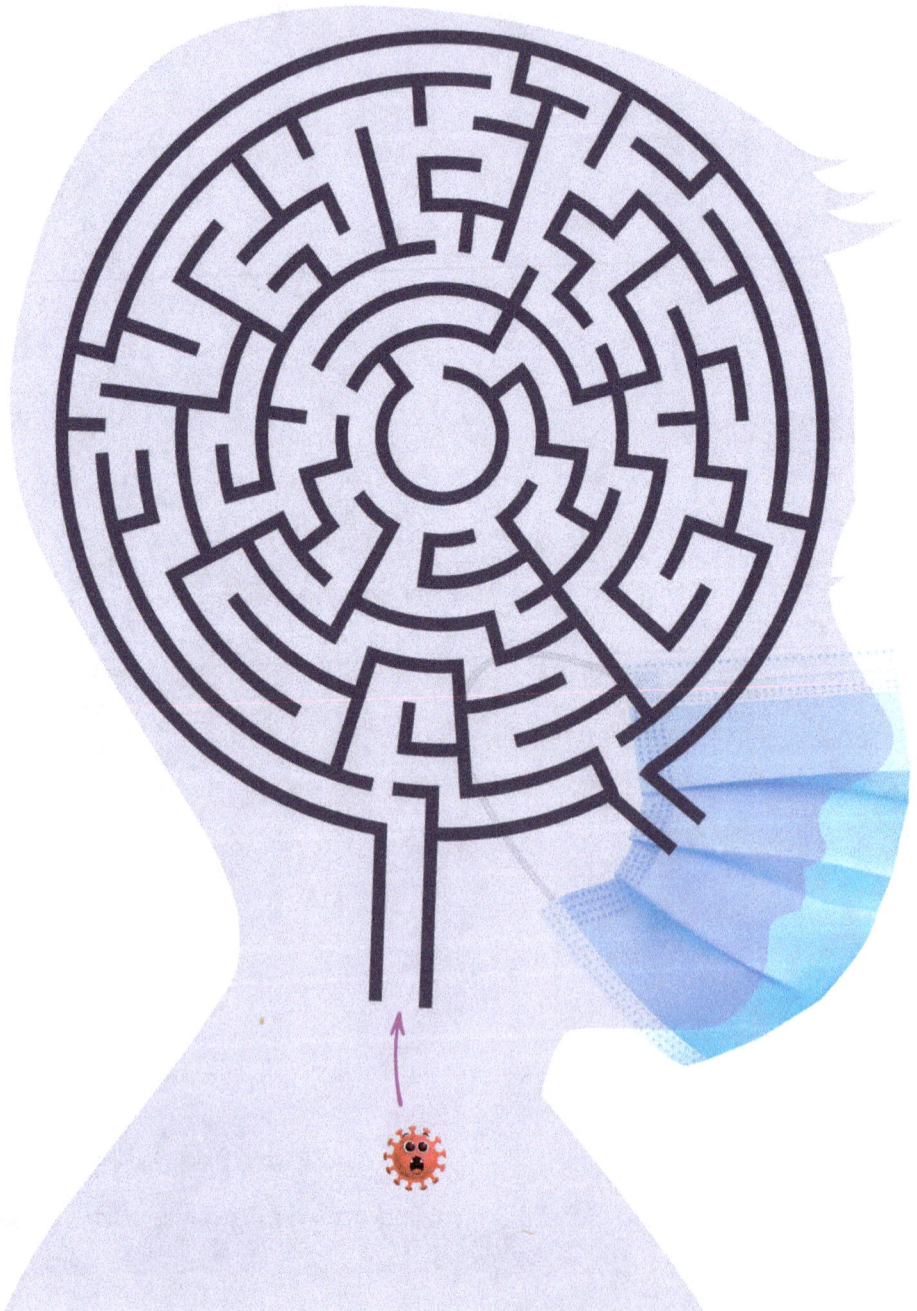

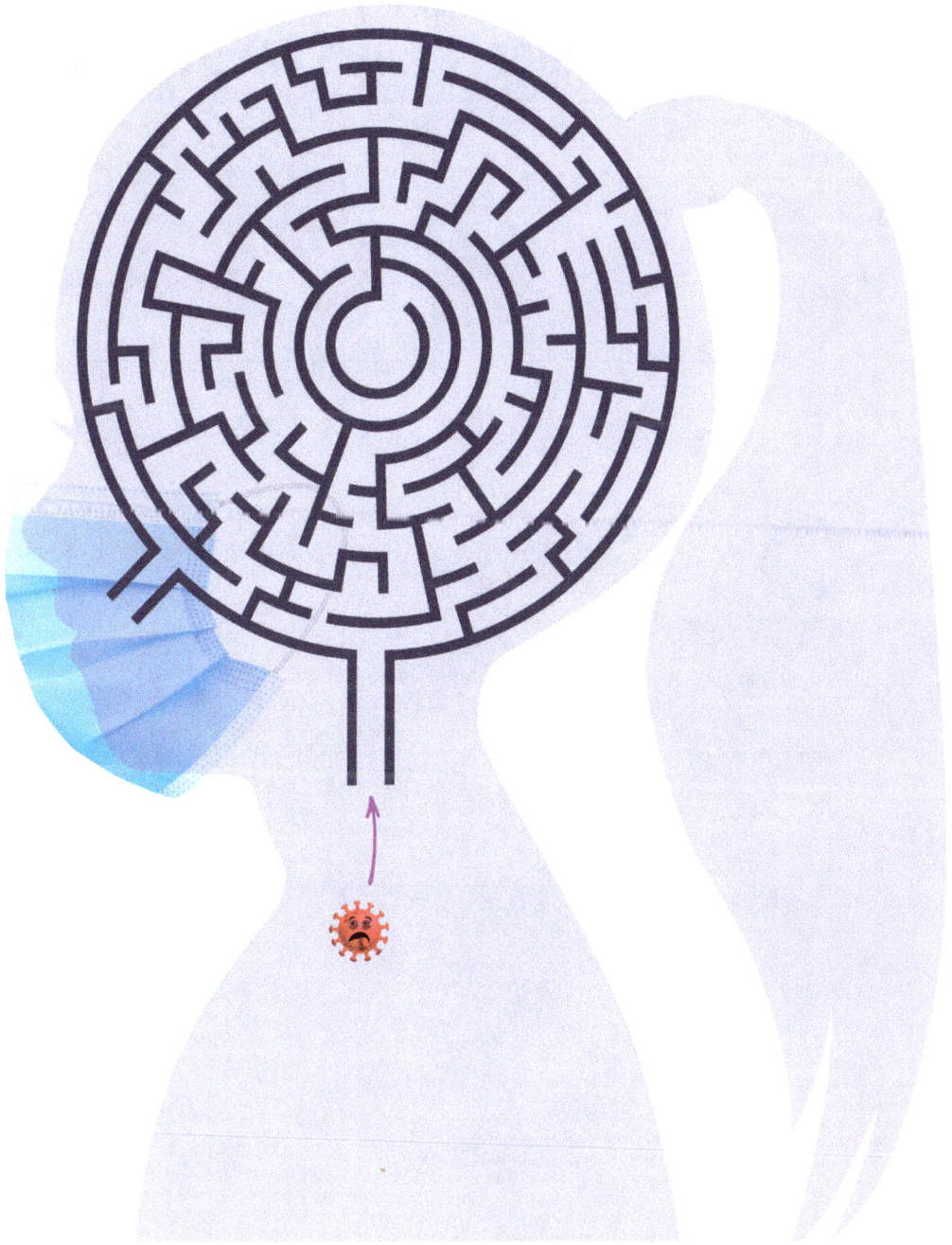

Coronavirus travels on tiny airborne drops that come out of our noses and mouths when we speak or cough. Masks catch many of these and protect other people.

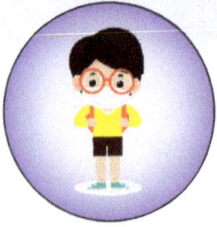

WHY SHOULDN'T I HUG MY friends or SHAKE OTHER PEOPLE'S HANDS?

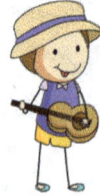

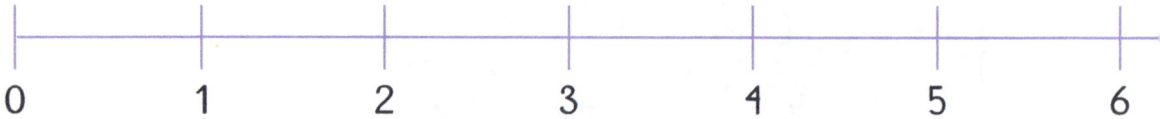

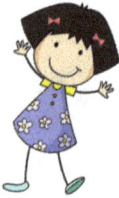

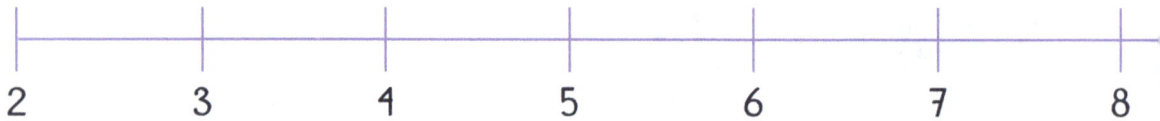

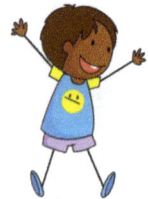

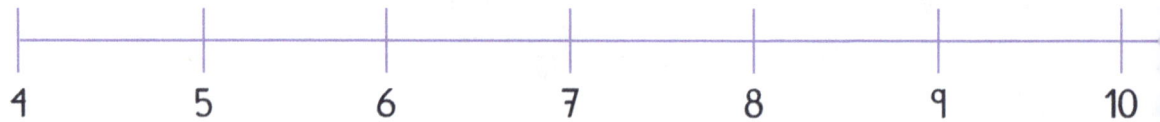

0	1	2	3	4	5	6

2	3	4	5	6	7	8

4	5	6	7	8	9	10

Count the steps between each pair of kids playing together and write the number in the Number Box. If the number is 6 or more, color the Number Box green for **GO**. If the number is 5 or less, color the Number Box red for **STOP**.

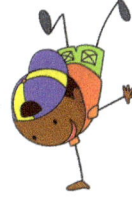

Number Box

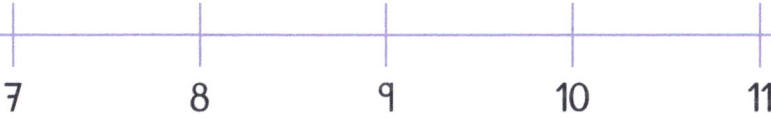

7　　8　　9　　10　　11

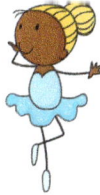

Number Box

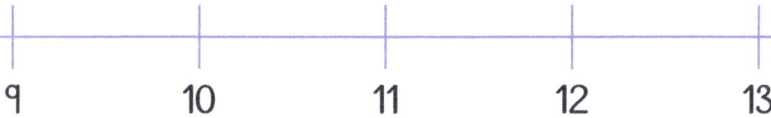

9　　10　　11　　12　　13

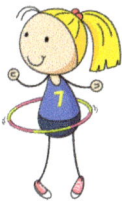

Number Box

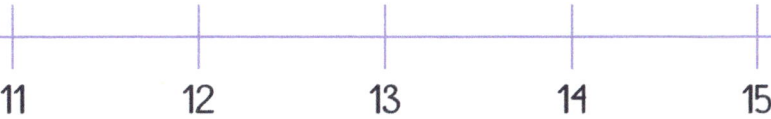

11　　12　　13　　14　　15

Physical contact with others creates a shorter journey with fewer obstacles for a traveling virus, making it easier to spread from one person to another.

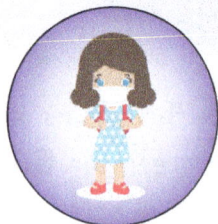

WHY SHOULDN'T WE SHARE OUR WRITING UTENSILS AND OTHER MATERIALS?

As the days pass by, write the subtraction problem answer on the blank line in the number sentence and draw the number of viruses left on the objects.

Monday

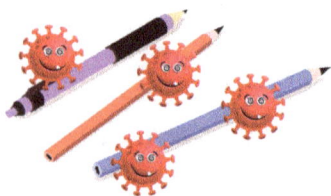

4

Tuesday

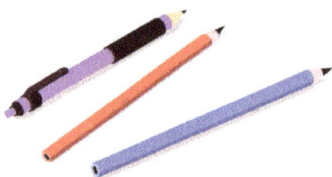

4 - 1 = ___

Wednesday

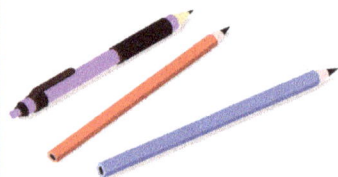

3 - 1 = ___

Thursday

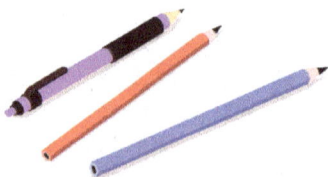

2 - 1 = ___

Friday

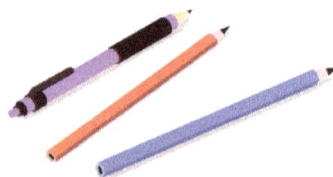

1 - 1 = ___

Saturday	Sunday	Monday

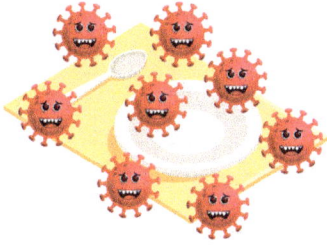

8

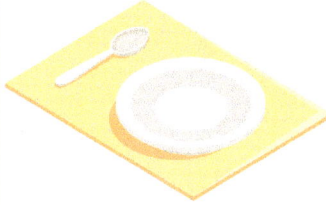

8 - 2 = ___

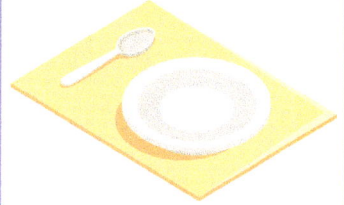

6 - 2 = ___

Tuesday	Wednesday

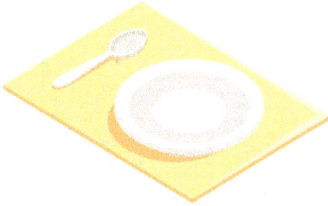

4 - 2 = ___

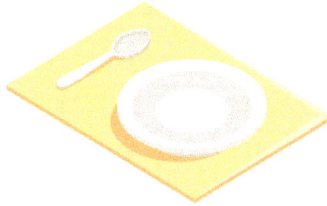

2 - 2 = ___

Coronavirus can live on spoons, pens and other objects for up to a few days. Sharing materials could spread the virus between students.

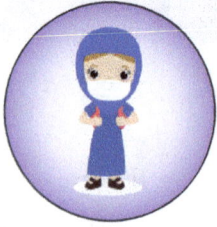

HOW COULD I GET SICK FROM TOUCHING MY FACE?

Fill in the number shapes with the colors below. Which parts are not colored?

1 → red
2 → orange
3 → yellow
4 → green
5 → blue
6 → purple
7 → pink
8 → brown
9 → black

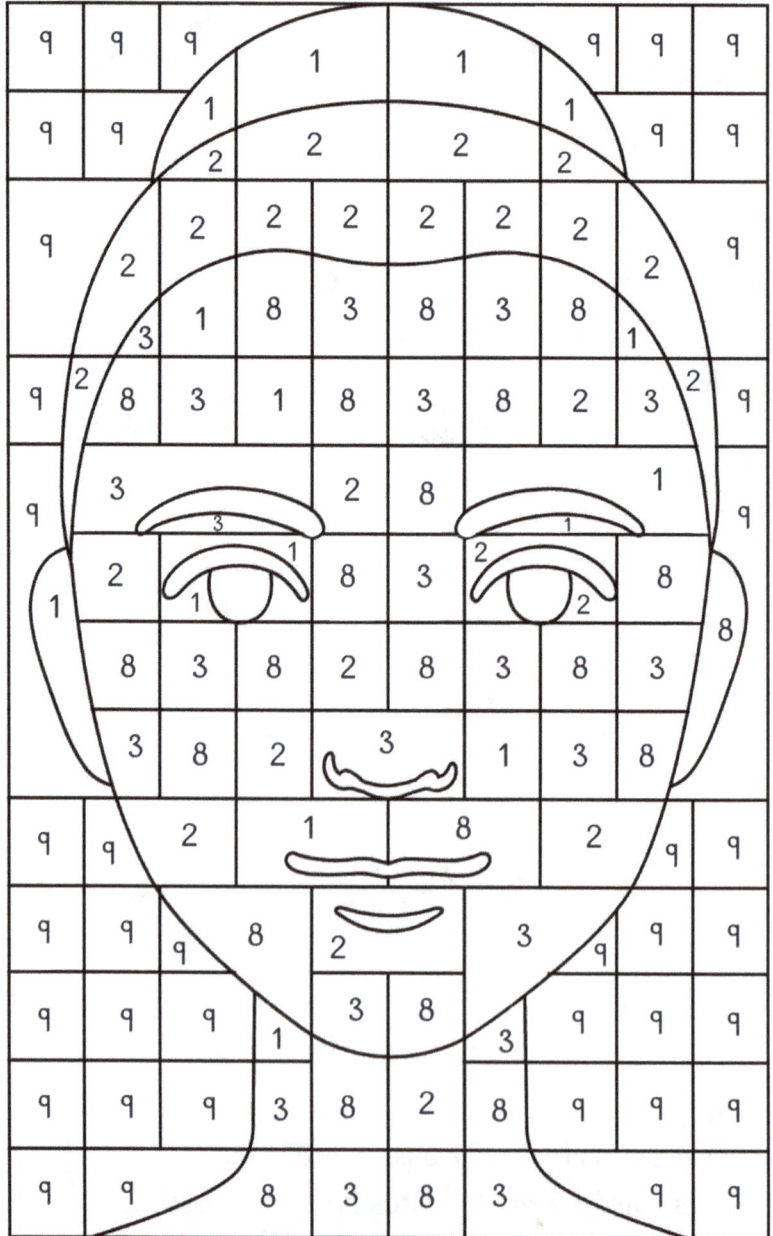

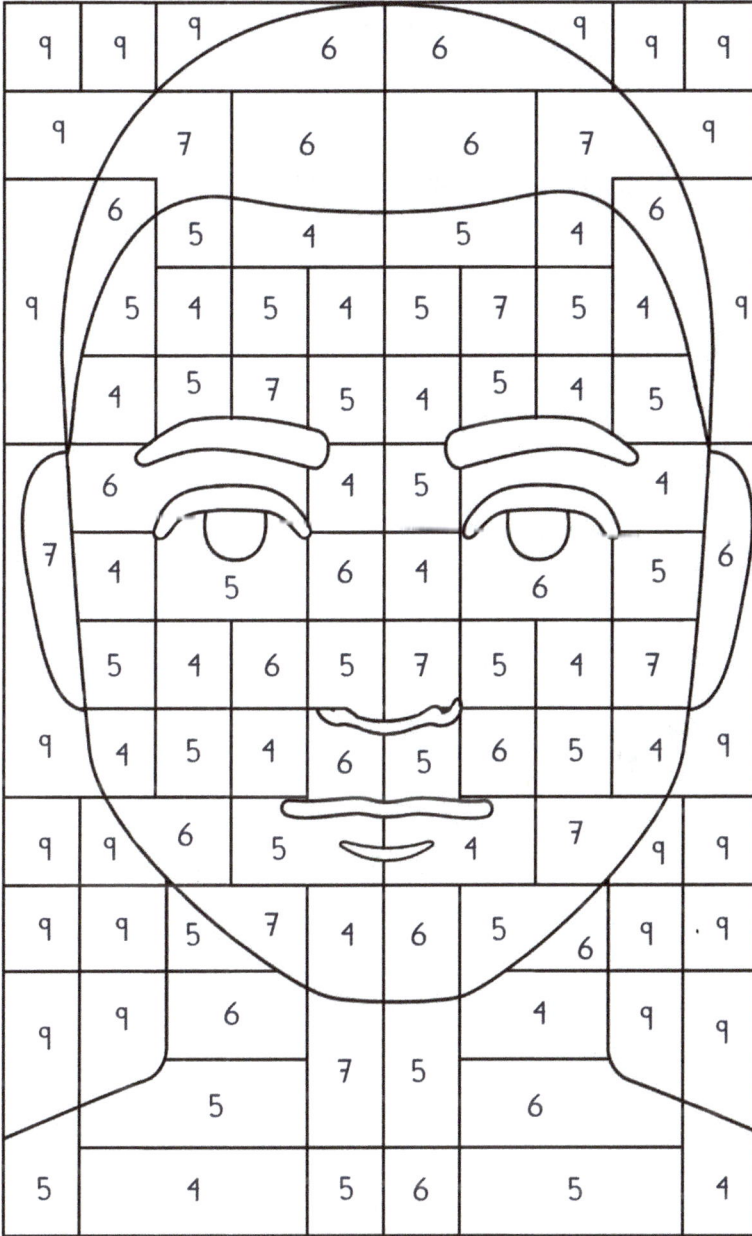

If you touch an infected surface and then touch your face, coronavirus can enter your body through your eyes, nose, or mouth like passing through an open window.

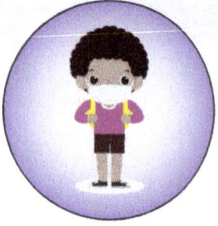

How Does Airing Out a Room Reduce the Risk of Getting Sick?

Count the number of droplets that have been blown away by the breeze and write the number down. Then cross out that many droplets inside the window.

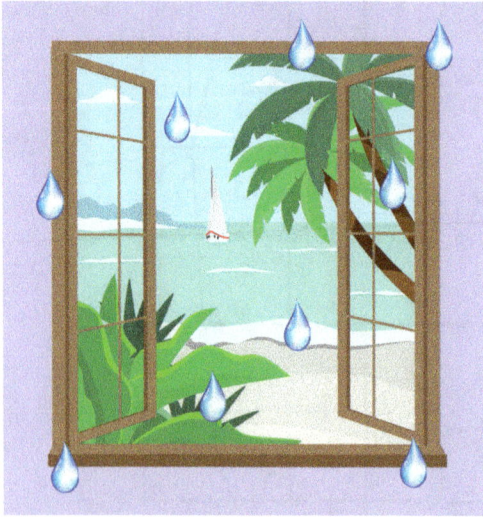

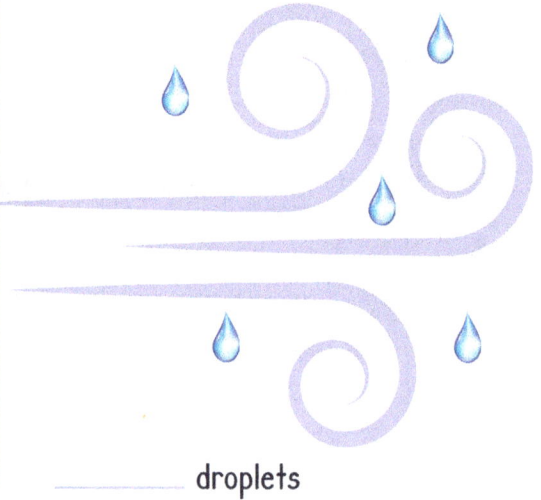

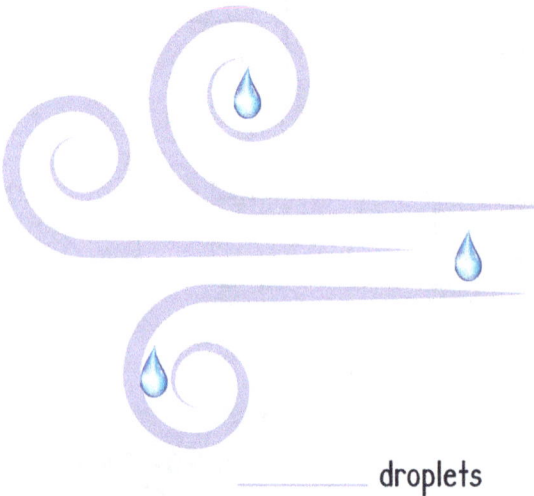

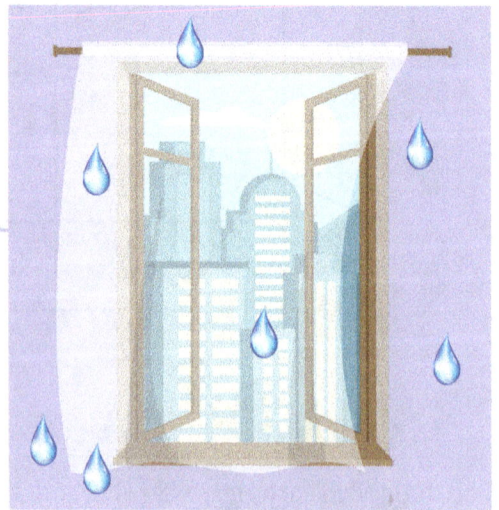

_____ droplets

_____ droplets

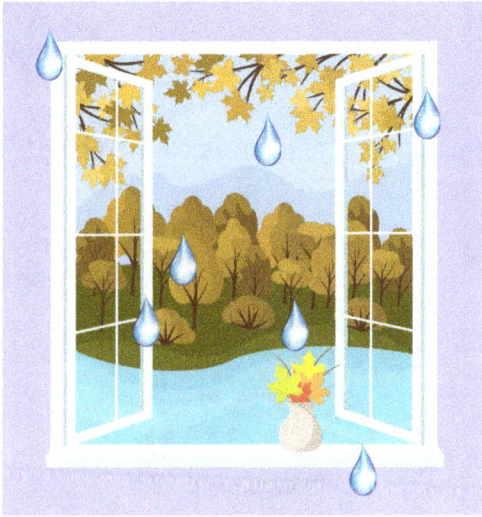

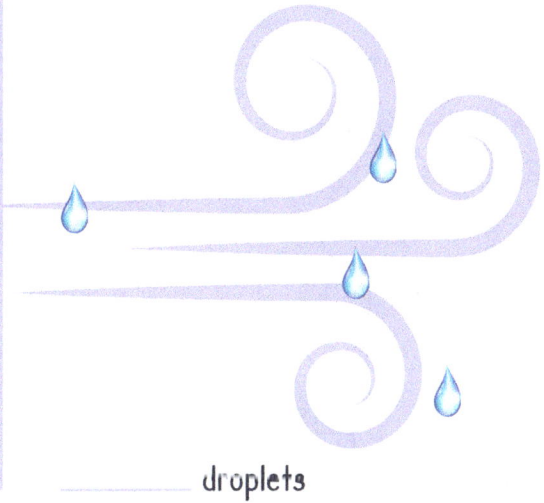

_____ droplets

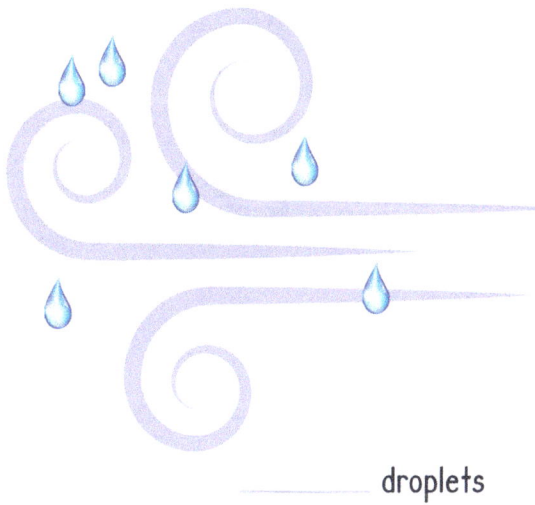

_____ droplets

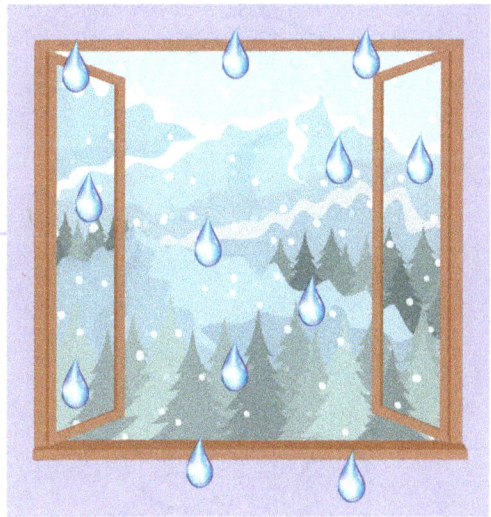

When a room has good ventilation, tiny droplets that we have exhaled from our lungs don't stay in the air as long.

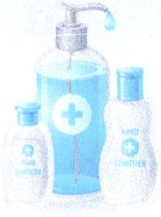

WHAT SHOULD I DO if I HAVE to COUGH or sneeze?

Color all the objects you might touch with your hands. Then circle all the objects you might touch with your elbow.

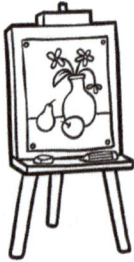

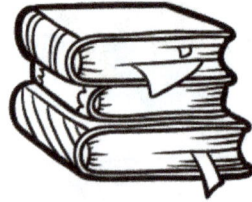

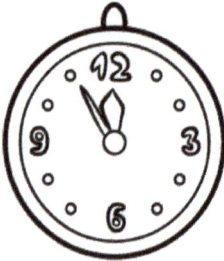

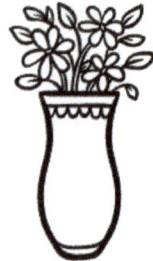

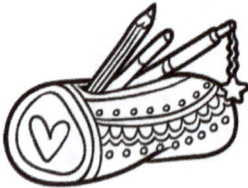

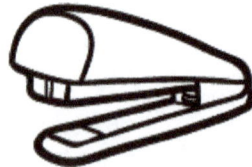

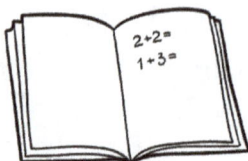

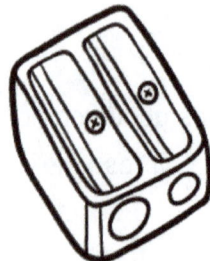

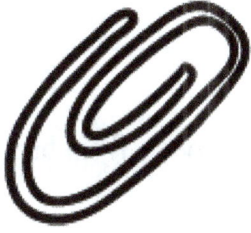

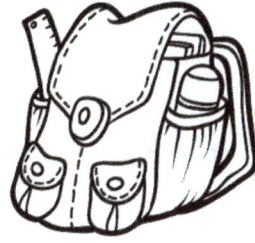

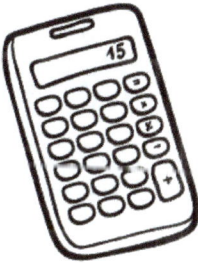

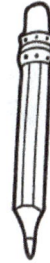

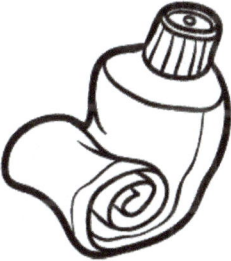

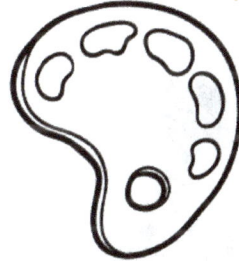

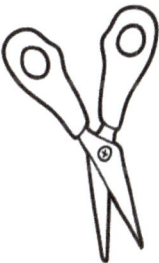

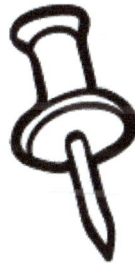

Using a tissue is best, but if you don't have a tissue, covering with your elbow is better than your hands because you touch more with your hands than your elbows.

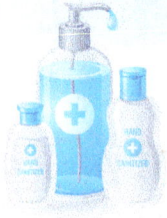

HOW SHOULD I WASH MY HANDS SO THEY'RE CLEAN ENOUGH?

Reorder and draw the hand washing steps on the next page from beginning to end.

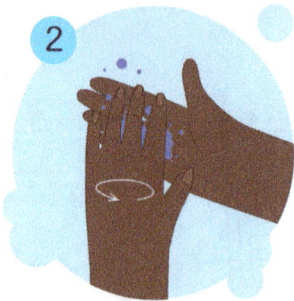

Rub palms.

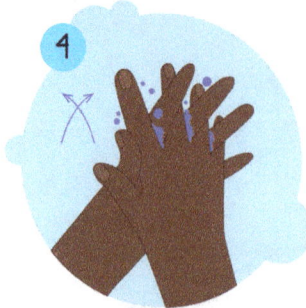

Lace fingers.

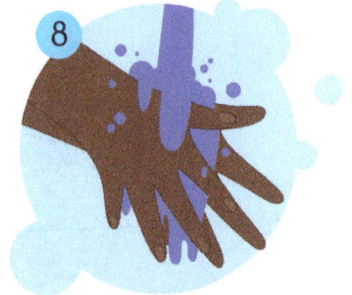

Rinse hands.

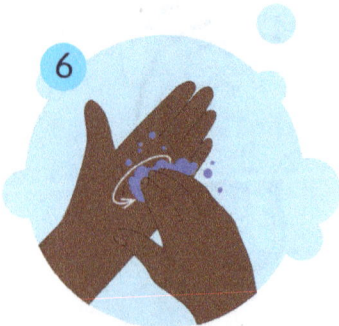

Swirl fingernails.

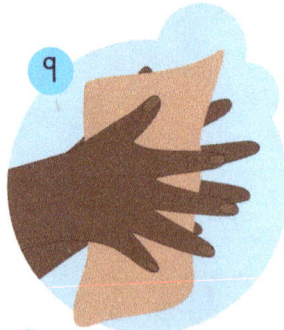

Towel dry.

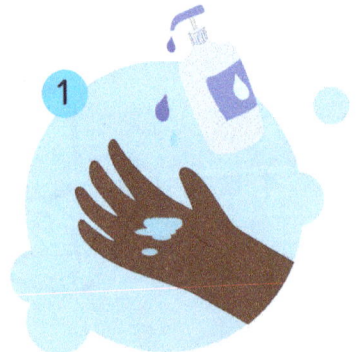

Use soap.

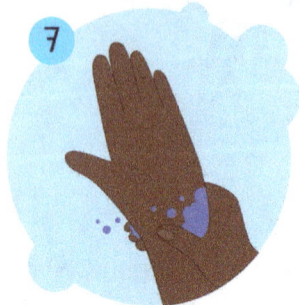

Clean wrists.

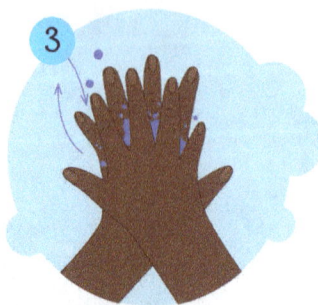

Scrub backs.

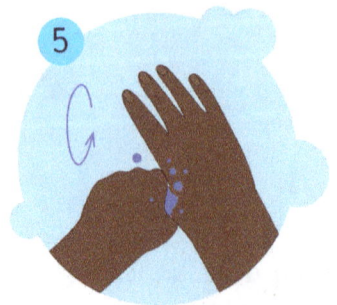

Polish thumbs.

Scrub your hands with soap and warm water for at least 20 seconds, rubbing the soap everywhere, including fingertips and the tops of your hands.

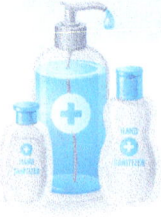

Does hand sanitizer work as well as washing with soap and water?

Trace your left hand on this page and your right hand on the next page. Then scribble out all the viruses on your hands with a blue "hand sanitizer" marker.

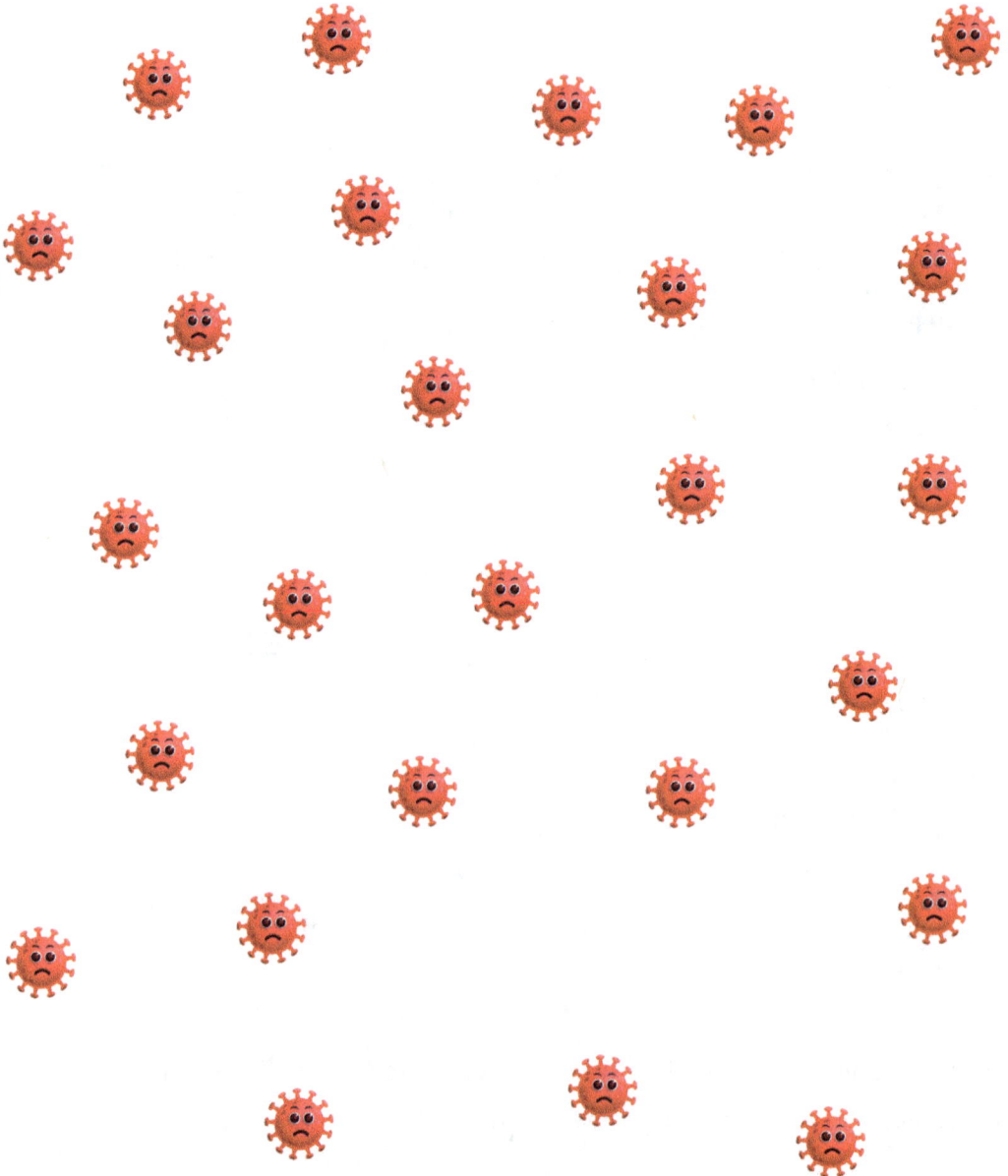

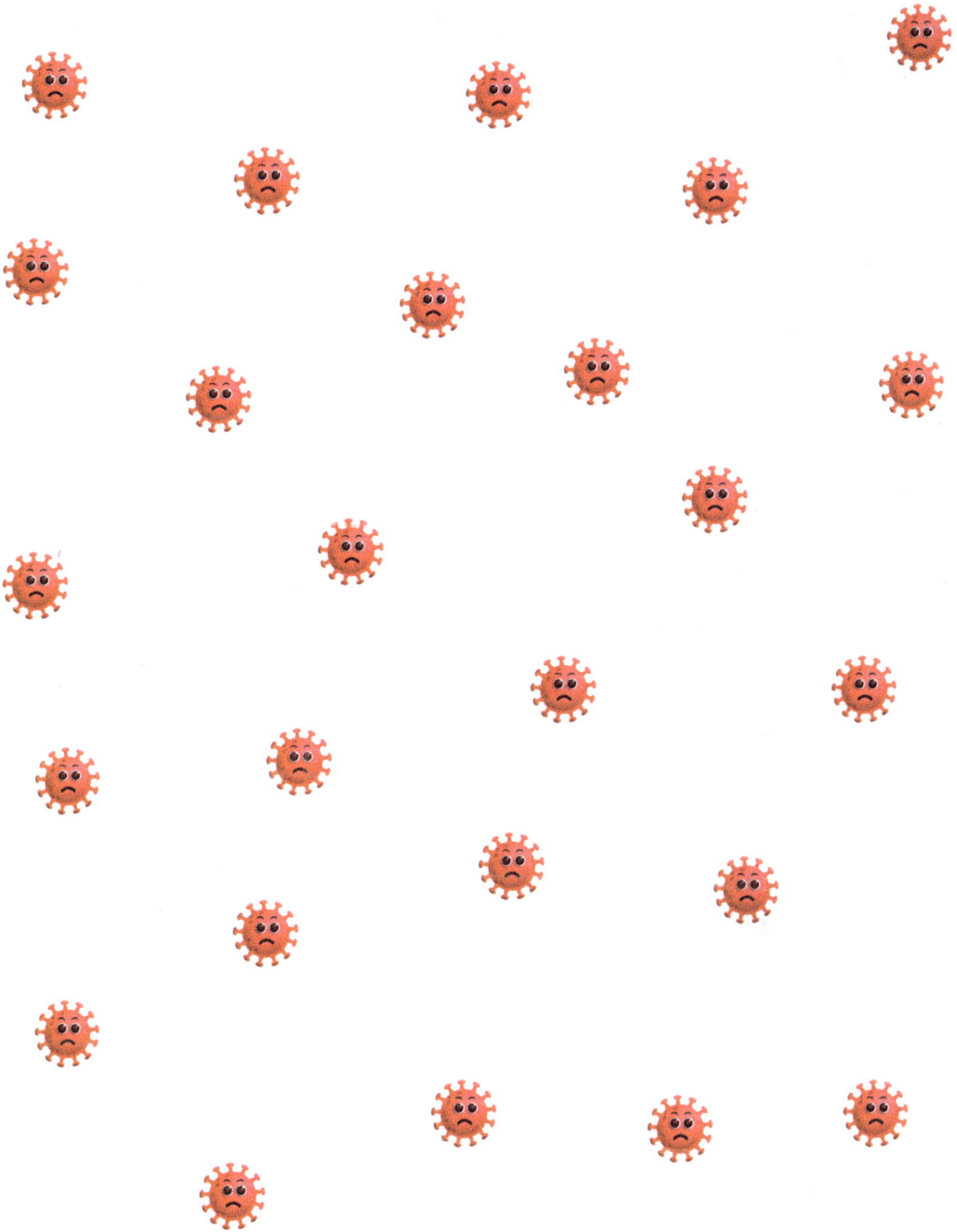

Washing hands with soap and water is best, but when it's not possible, sanitizer with 60% alcohol is helpful. Never put your fingers in your mouth after using sanitizer.

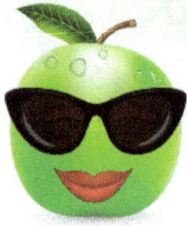

How does drinking water help my body fight viruses and sickness?

In each box, circle the child who drank the most water.

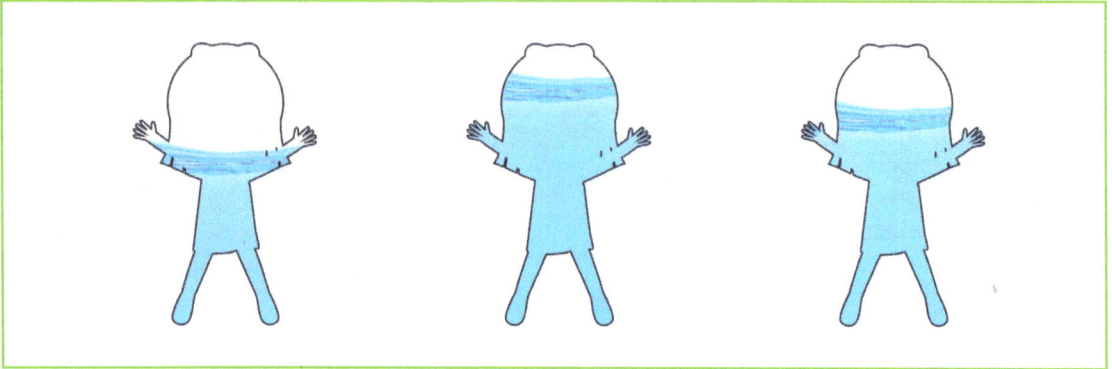

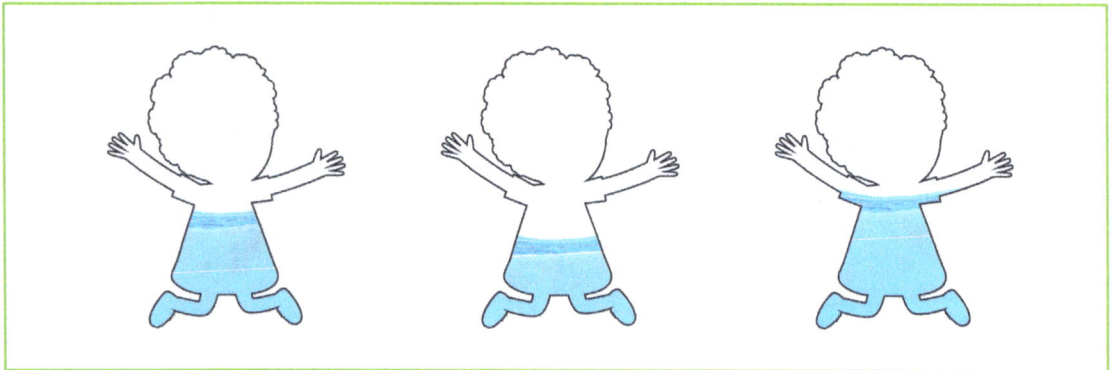

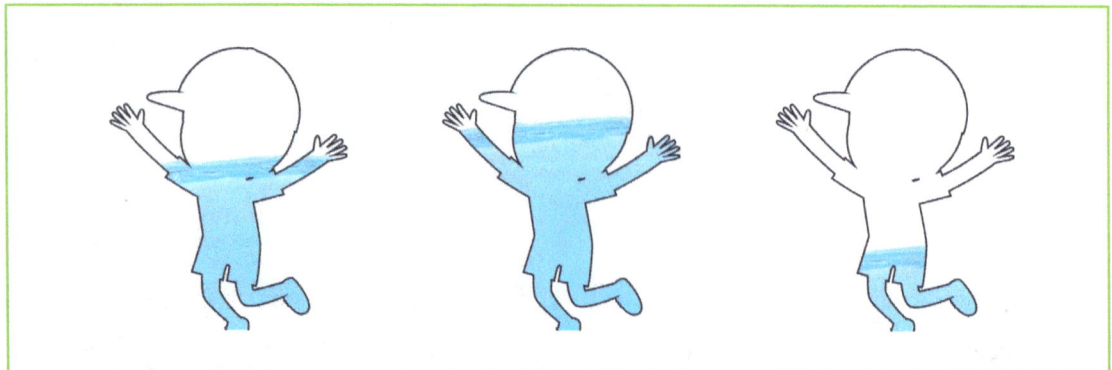

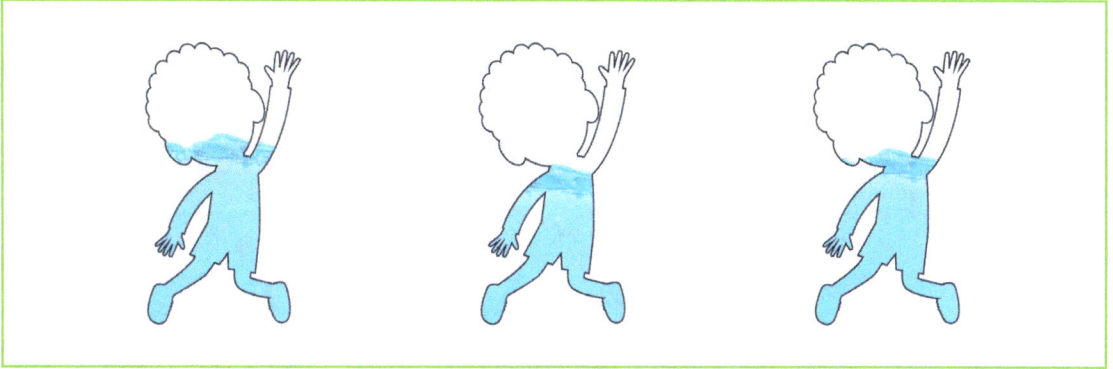

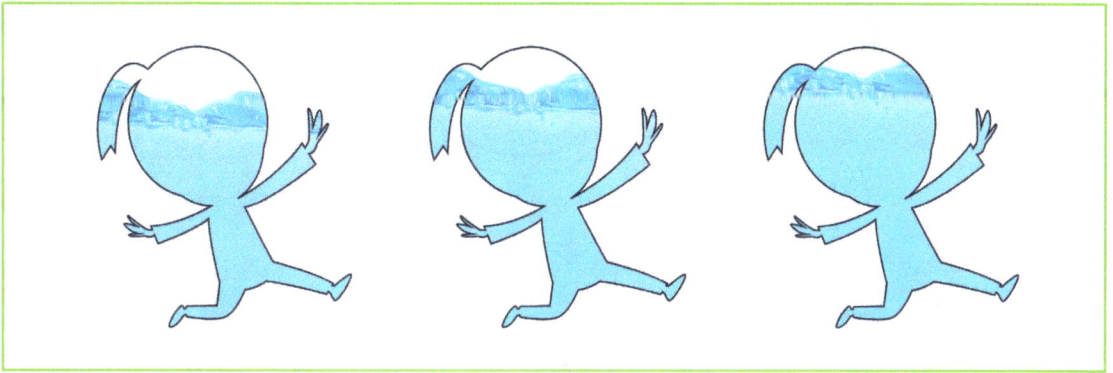

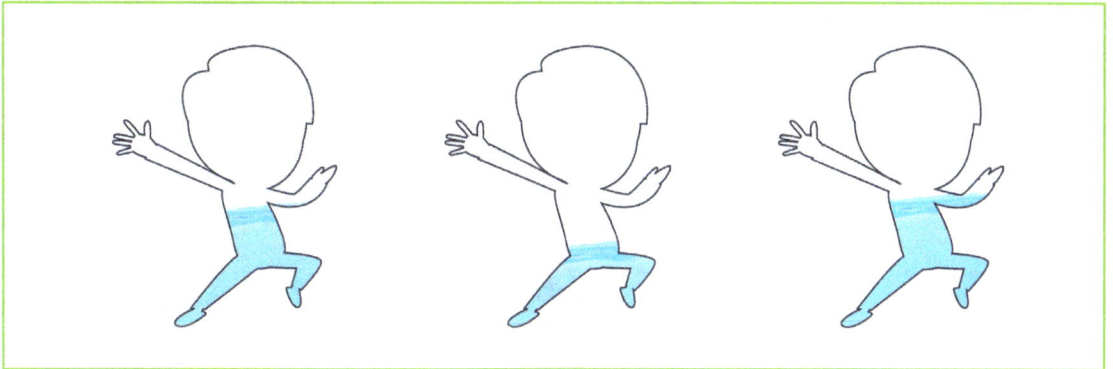

Water carries nutrients throughout your body and helps flush the garbage out. Depending on how big you are, you should drink up to 8 glasses a day.

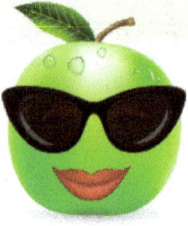

WHICH FOODS KEEP ME HEALTHY?

Color the foods that help keep you healthy and cross out the unhealthy foods.

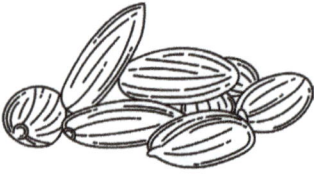

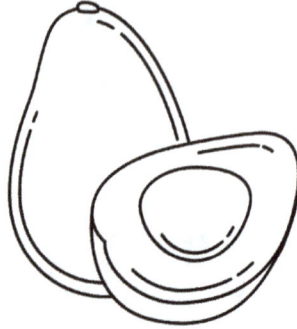

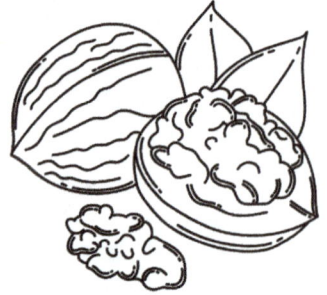

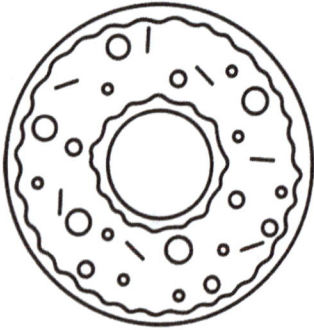

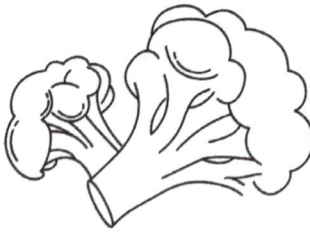

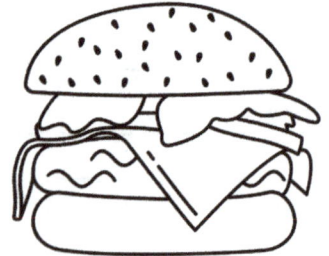

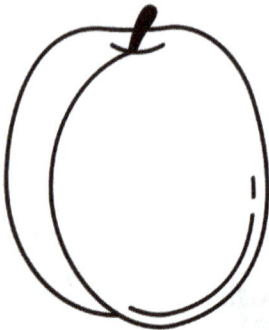

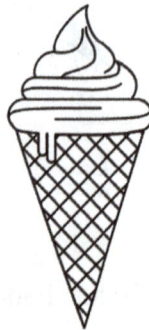

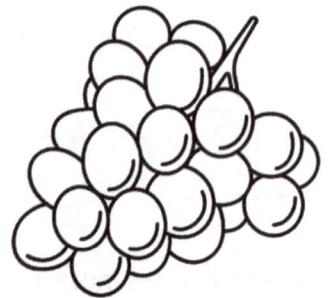

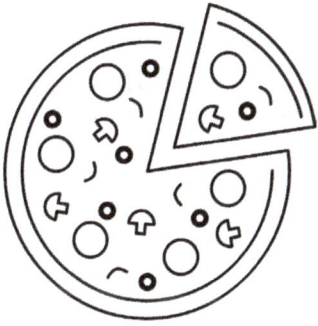

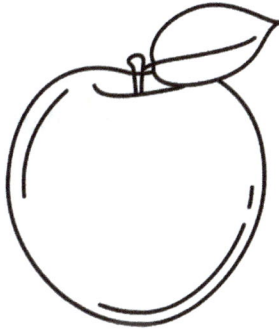

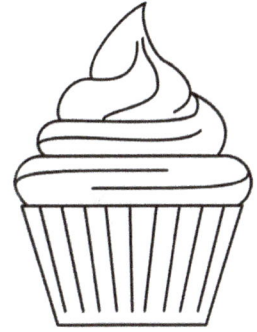

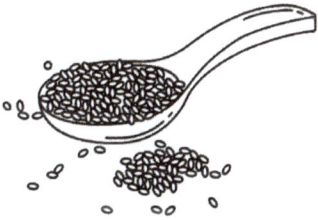

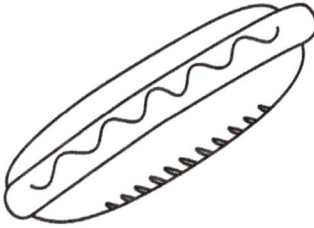

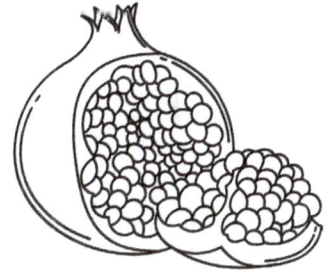

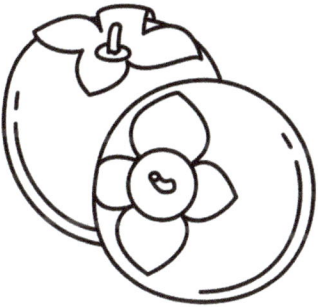

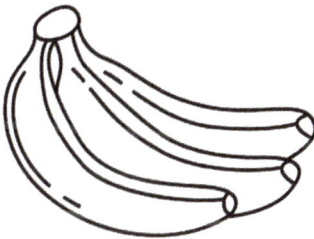

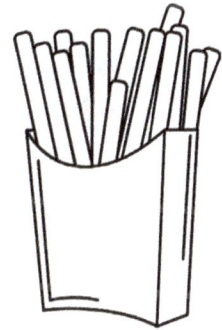

Some good foods for a strong immune system include fruits and vegetables, low-fat milk, seafood, seeds and nuts.

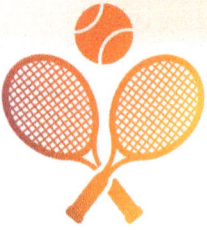

WHY are sports, exercise and other PHYSICAL activities good for me?

Write the shadow's letter next to its matching physical activity.

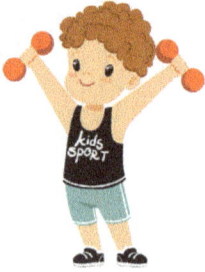

Shadow _____

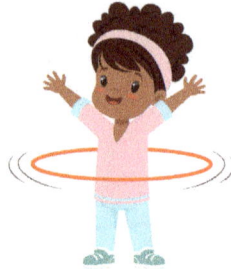

Shadow _____

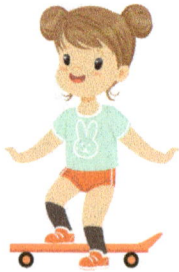

Shadow _____

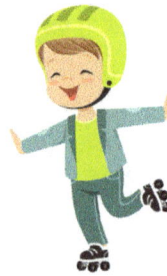

Shadow _____

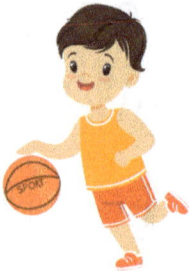

Shadow _____

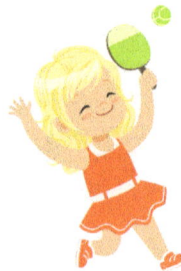

Shadow _____

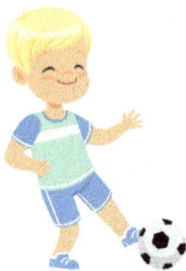

Shadow _____

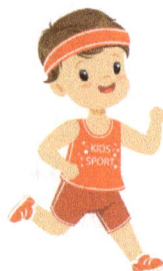

Shadow _____

A

B

C

D

E

F

G

H

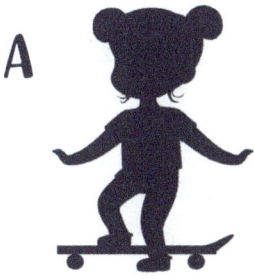

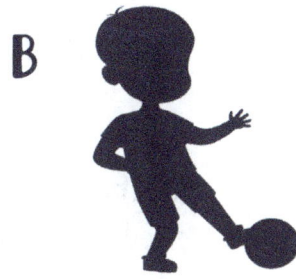

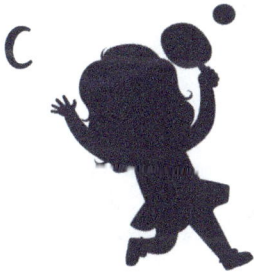

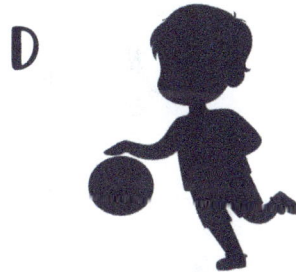

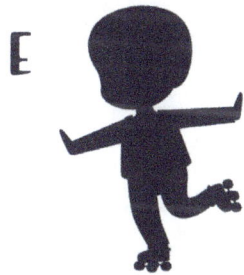

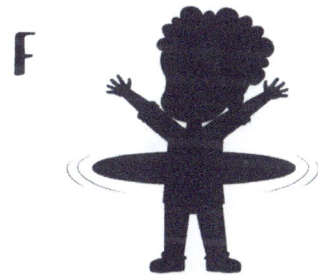

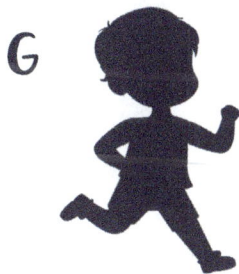

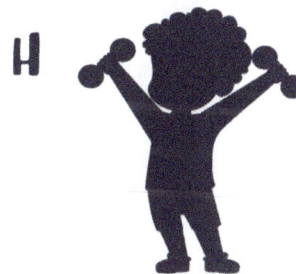

Regular physical activity helps your body fight sickness and disease.

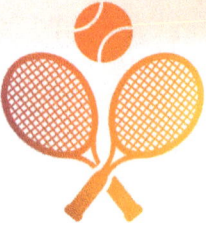

WHAT GAMES CAN I PLAY WITH MY FRIENDS IF I HAVE TO KEEP SOCIAL DISTANCE?

In every orange circle, draw either a green ✓ for games kids can play from a safe distance apart or a red X for those where children play too closely together.

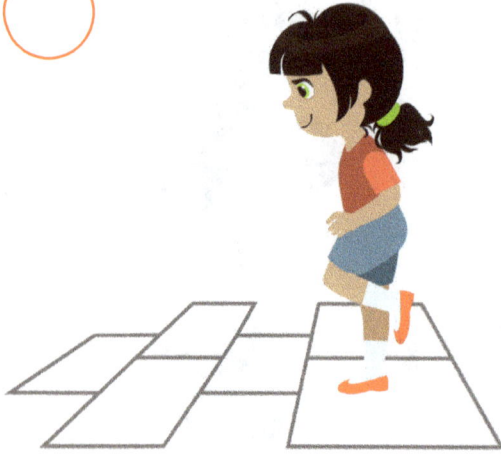

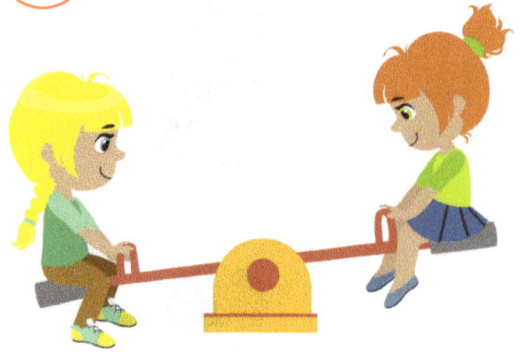

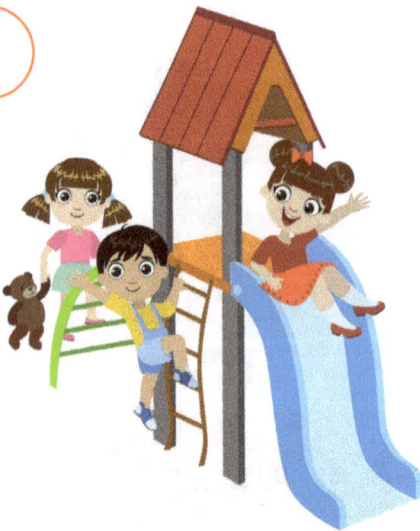

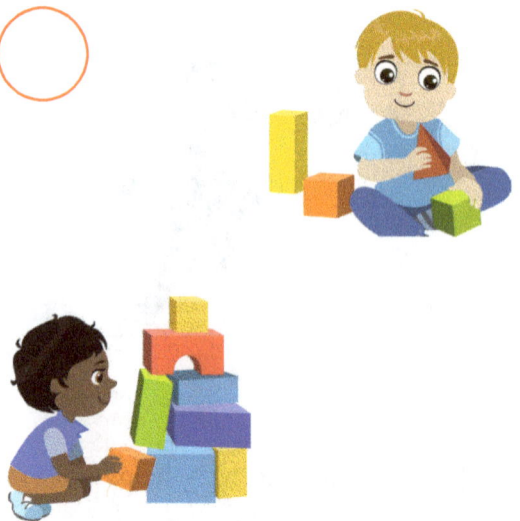

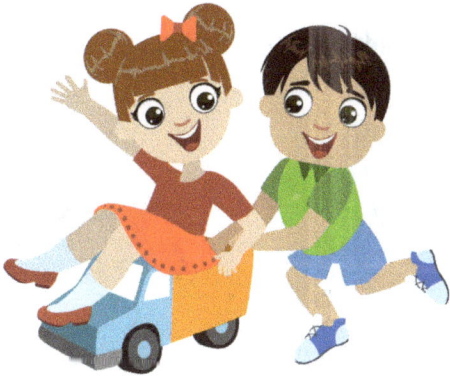

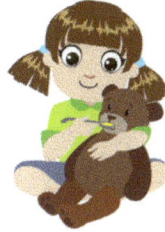

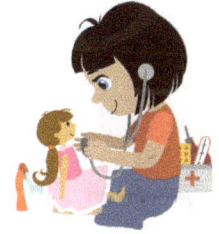

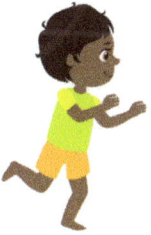

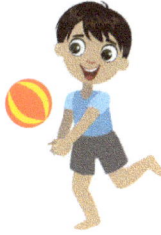

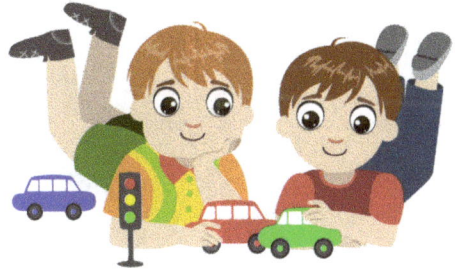

Safe games include tennis, ping pong, four-square and safe versions of soccer, baseball and other non-contact sports. Games to avoid are tag, wrestling, or capture.

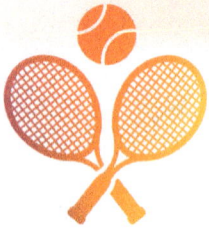

HOW MUCH SLEEP SHOULD I GET EVERY NIGHT TO STAY HEALTHY?

Draw lines between matching shapes to send the kids to their beds.

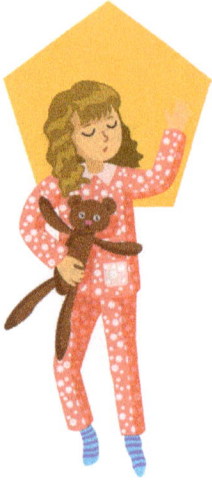

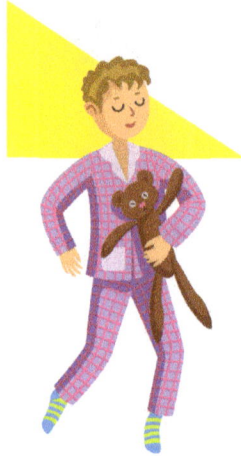

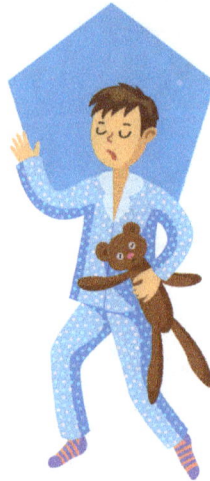

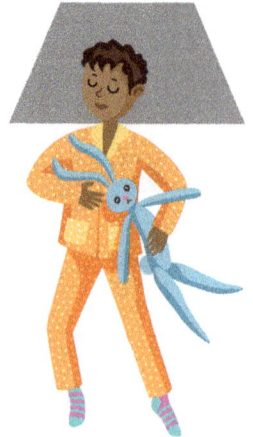

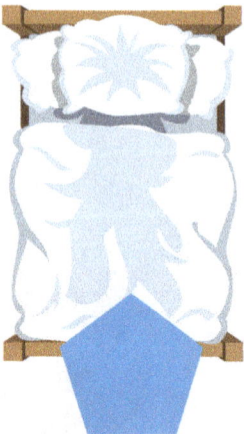

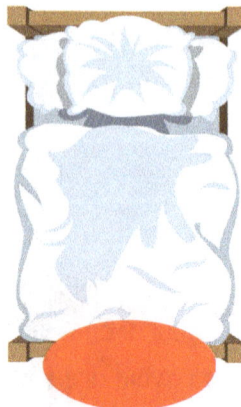

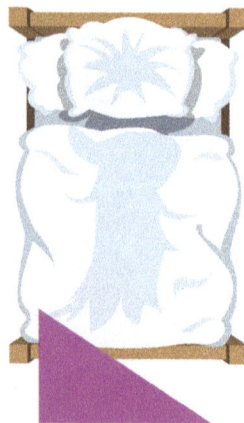

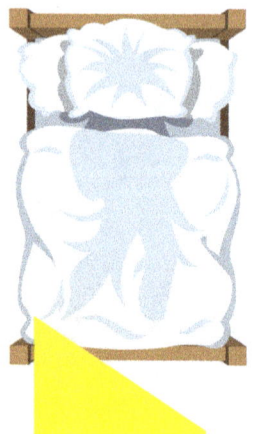

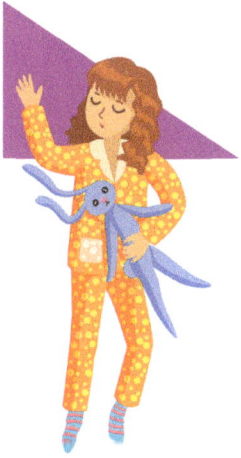

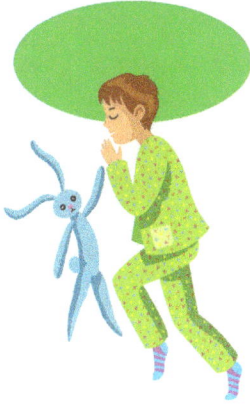

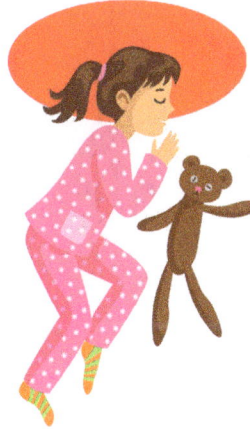

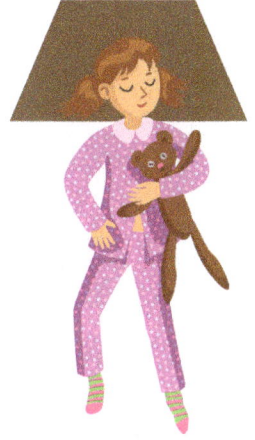

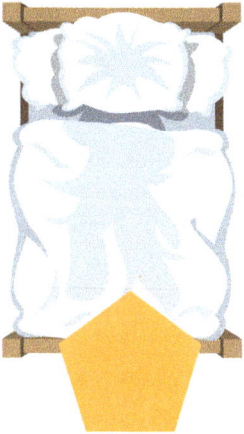

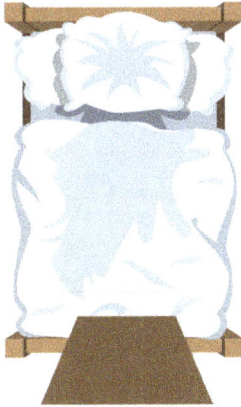

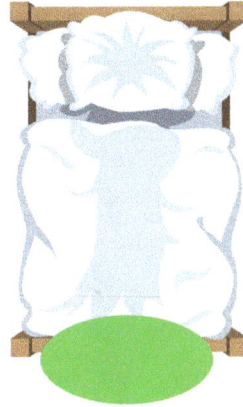

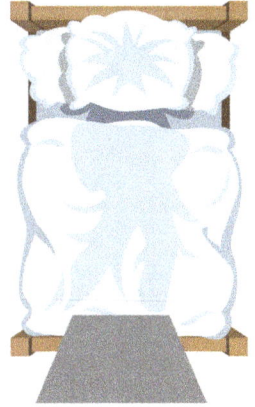

While you sleep your body has a chance to recharge, keeping your immune and other systems strong. Depending on your age and size, you should get 8-11 hours of sleep.